Better Health with (Mostly) Chinese Herbs and Foods

健康

Albert Y. Leung, Ph.D.
Pharmacognosist
Consultant in Natural Products

Photographs by Stephen Foster
Book Design by Marion Gold

AYSL Corporation
Glen Rock, New Jersey

Published in the United States of America
by AYSL Corporation
P.O. Box 181, Glen Rock, NJ 07452

Printed in Canada

10 9 8 7 6 5 4 3 2 1

Library of Congress Cataloging-in-Publication Data

Leung, Albert Y.
Better Health with (Mostly) Chinese Herbs and Foods

Bibliography: p.
Includes index.
1. Herbs — Therapeutic use. 2. Materia medica, Vegetable — China. 3. Medicine, Chinese — Formulae, receipts, prescriptions. 4. Medicine, Chinese — History. I. Title.

RM666.H33L48 1995 615′.321 94-96790
ISBN 0-9634979-1-X CIP

To my wife Barbara and
our grown daughters Amy and Camille.

PREFACE

When my *Encyclopedia of Common Natural Ingredients Used in Food, Drugs and Cosmetics* (Wiley, 1980) was first published fifteen years ago, there were few English scientific books on botanicals. Since that time, many books on this subject have appeared. Now, there is no longer a vacuum of scientific information on herbs. Accurate information on herbs can be readily obtained through two nonprofit organizations, the Herb Research Foundation and the American Botanical Council. They also jointly publish the *HerbalGram*, which in my opinion is the most accurate and impartial publication on herbs. Nevertheless, along with these new developments in recent years comes the potential danger of abandoning true-and-tried healing methods based on herbs, opting instead for more single-chemical toxic drugs that have increasingly been causing more and more problems for those who use them. Let me remind you, despite claims by the medical and drug establishments, medicine is not strictly a science, because a huge variable, our body, consisting of myriads of different types of experimentally uncontrollable tissues and cells, is ignored. All the medical and drug research on humans so far has been conducted under the assumption that you and I are the same. But you and I know we definitely are not! No magic of medical statistics can change that!

Most scientific research and publications on medicinal herbs treat these herbs as if they only exist to provide single-chemical drugs, eventually to be synthesized and marketed by drug companies. The researchers and authors have forgotten that many of these herbs are part of our diet and have been safely and effectively used for millennia to better our health and to prevent illnesses. Many of these herbs are good as they are in their natural form and should not be turned into single-chemical drugs that are frequently toxic and don't work as well. We need to not lose sight of a basic principle of many traditional formulas: the efficacy is dependent on the combination of ingredients contained in the native herbs, not on single compounds. In fact, the relatively low incidence of side reactions attributed to traditional medicines is frequently the result of certain potentially toxic ingredients being ameliorated by other ingredients present. While single-chemical drugs are sometimes necessary for certain illnesses, even these illnesses can benefit from traditional herbs and foods. For those interested in single-chemical drugs from herbs, there are already some excellent drug-oriented books on this subject, notably ones by Professor Varro Tyler.[1,2] What we need are books that offer another viewpoint. It is for this reason that I have written *Better Health with (Mostly) Chinese Herbs and Foods.* I hope this book will incite you to reevaluate your thinking towards modern single-chemical drugs and traditional herbs, leading to a change of health habits and hopefully a healthier life with more herbs/foods and less toxic modern drugs.

Most of the information on Chinese herbs in this book comes from my own library and database on Chinese herbal medicine, which include all major traditional Chinese herbals and over sixty modern Chinese journals on this subject. Much of the information on Chinese herbs in the book is available in English for the first time. For interested scientists and professionals, technical data on these herbs are summarized in my revised *Encyclopedia* which will be available in August, 1995.

I wish to thank the many friends and colleagues who had urged me to write this book. Special thanks go to: Marion Gold for designing the book, including the cover, and for utilizing his desktop publishing skills to considerably speed up the production of this book; and Steven Foster for supplying the exquisite photographs.

Lastly, I also wish to thank my wife Barbara and our older daughter Amy for reviewing the manuscript and offering some very valuable comments.

References

1. Tyler, V.E. 1987. *The New Honest Herbal.* George F. Stickley Co. Philadelphia, PA.

2. Tyler, V.E. 1994. *Herbs of Choice - The Therapeutic Use of Phytomedicinals.* Pharmaceutical Products Press. Binghamton, N.Y.

Better Health with (Mostly) CHINESE HERBS & FOODS

Much has been written about herbs. But what *is* an herb? In botanical terms, an herb is a plant that does not have a woody stem above ground as do trees and shrubs. Thus, mint, ginger, daisy, celery and watercress are herbs. Strictly speaking, the banana "tree" is also an herb — a giant herb — because although it may attain a height of fifteen to twenty feet, it does not have a woody stem.

For everyday usage, however, an herb can be defined as in *Webster's Dictionary*, *i.e.*, "a plant or plant part used for its culinary, flavoring and medicinal qualities." So, an herb can be a spice or condiment, a medicine, or a food (vegetable, fruit, grain or nut). We normally think of an herb as either one of the former, but rarely as a food. In this book, I will introduce you to some commonly used herbs that have been safely used for hundreds to thousands of years as spices, medicines and foods.

By "commonly used" I don't mean herbs that only Westerners consider as common, such as celery, mint, rosemary and thyme. I also consider as common some herbs and foods used by hundreds of millions of people of other cultures, especially Chinese and East Indian, where use history is normally measured by millennia or centuries and not by generations or decades. America (both Canada and the United States) is an immigrant society, with the American Indians being the only true natives. As immigrants, we have brought with us numerous aspects of our diverse cultures. Among the most important are our foods, herbs and healing methods. We Americans pride ourselves in our diversified racial, ethnic and cultural backgrounds. Without those unique qualities, we would simply be an Anglo, an African, a Latin, a Chinese, a Japanese, a

Scandinavian or whatever, and not even a true one at that.

Many, however, have forgotten this fact. They consider themselves more American than others just because (perhaps) they arrived here a few generations earlier, or are of a different culture. Without having any understanding or even a knowledge of our country's true heritage, they look down upon the cultural practices of their fellow Americans.

This is especially true in the realm of ethnic medicines. I can't speak for other ethnic groups because I am not familiar enough with their medical practices. But I can certainly comment on how Chinese herbal medicine is being treated in America, especially in the United States.

The Chinese healing system (traditional medicine, herbal medicine, acupuncture, massage, moxibition, *qi gong*, etc.) has been around for several thousand years, and has been used by billions of people safely and effectively for all these years. Even though its terminology may be "out-of-date" and often strange, it is *definitely* a legitimate health care system. Anyone will agree with me if he or she has taken the time to look into it. Yet, bureaucrats and some politically appointed officials in our government, without having any knowledge or understanding of traditional Chinese medicine whatsoever, are trying to restrict its practice, especially in the herbal area. What they don't know or understand they find easy to simply ban. I don't think it is simply an issue of the healing system itself, but rather a cultural and economic issue.

The bureaucrats may argue that they don't have enough safety data to allow certain herbs or formulas to be used in our foods or as medicines for general distribution. Yet they never bother to look into the matter objectively. Since the bureaucrats in charge are mostly from the same club whose members are from the drug industry and the conventional medical establishment, there is no need to look into an insignificant (in their thinking) and non-profitable (for them) system like Chinese herbal medicine or other ethnic medicines. Their attempt, if successful, would deny many of us the freedom of choice in taking care of our health. We don't want to be ill — nor be rendered more ill — by our "modern" medical (sick-care) system. Rather, we want to avoid modern drugs and to stay healthy with herbs and foods of our choice, which have been safely and beneficially used for centuries.

Well, then, why do we *use* herbs? Apart from the most obvious reason (as a spice or condiment), herbs are frequently used either as foods or as medicines. Often, in fact, there is a very fine line that separates the two. An herb can be a food or a medicine solely depending on how it is used. Take watercress as an example. It is definitely a food when normally consumed as a vegetable or salad. But if eaten with therapeutic intentions, watercress can be regarded as a medicine, such as for soothing the lungs. Frequently, we are not aware that many of our foods and spices are also time-honored medicines. These are some of the herbs that have sustained the human species and maintained its health for millennia.

• • •

In BETTER HEALTH WITH (MOSTLY) CHINESE HERBS & FOODS, I have chosen sixty herbs and foods to help better your health. They do not include herbs that are primarily medicines which do not have a food use history, or those that require considerable caution in their use. The selected herbs and foods are meant to supply certain unconventional nutrients which may be missing in our modern diets. The actions of these food herbs are mild and tend to help the body balance itself and correct any problems resulting from an imbalance. Perhaps that is the reason why most tonic herbs and foods have multiple uses, some of which on the surface may not seem to have any relationship to one another. But if the conditions are due to deficiency of certain not-yet-recognized nutrients that affect our body universally at a cellular level, correcting this deficiency would have extensive health ramifications. Nevertheless, even with foods, one of the most important rules in partaking is moderation. If you observe this rule, you will enjoy the benefits of these herbal foods with minimal unpleasant consequences.

Why do we *need* herbs? The answer can be academic. Using herbs is a very personal thing. If you are happy and "healthy" living in this modern world of ours, with its advanced technology and convenient foods, you might not think you need herbs. Our society has conditioned us to regard routinely taking government-approved drugs as a normal thing to do. Even though you may suffer from headaches (suppressed by these drugs) or nervousness (also drug-suppressed) or other drug-suppressed or induced (and suppressed) conditions, you may consider yourself basically healthy. After all, the way we have grown up with drug advertisements everywhere, everyone must be taking a lot of drugs. You have been conditioned to believe there is a pill for every little ache or pain or up or down that you may experience. And you must be "quite healthy" because you are *only* taking one or two of these drugs — drugs our government tells us are safe — which are heavily promoted by the drug industry and mandated by our government as the only medicines to take if we want to be healthy. In fact, you may well be "healthy" in a way you have known best or been conditioned to accept as a healthy state.

Sadly, however, you may not truly be healthy, and may not know what true health is. I like to give this analogy:

> If one has grown up eating chop suey, and believing that this is genuine Chinese cuisine, one is probably perfectly happy with chop suey. There is no need or reason for one to think or feel otherwise. The same is true with one's health. Why

should you feel you are unhealthy if you have not had a chance to experience true health?

A lot of our everyday aches and pains are caused by the drugs we take and the environments in which we live. Add to these the unhealthy foods we eat, and most of us probably never feel one hundred percent healthy, even though we might believe we are.

The United States is considered the most advanced in medical and drug research in the world. Yet we are shamefully the worst in infant mortality rates among developed nations, and our citizens are not healthier than those of countries like China, whose health care system our health providers frown upon. Our problem is obviously not that we lack drugs or advanced medical and surgical technology. Our problem is that we have *too much* of both, as well as *too much* financial incentive for those in control to freely dispense them. Our health care system has somehow evolved into its current state, which can best be described as a "sick-care" system.

In the on-going health care debate, the "experts" have totally missed the point. Or have they? After all, who will be reaping the most financial benefits? Not you and I. It is a system in which there is no incentive for the major health care providers (especially drug manufacturers and medical doctors) to keep us healthy, because there are many more financial rewards by keeping us ill. Just take a look around and you will see what I mean. There are drug ads everywhere, conditioning us early on in our life to take drugs (synthetic, toxic drugs with no more than several decades' "safe" history of use) for even minor conditions that don't require drugs to resolve. The more drugs we are enticed to take, the healthier drug industry profits become.

Doctors also benefit because they get a cut of these profits through visitation and prescription fees, and some even receive special perks from drug companies for prescribing these drugs. The bureaucrats and government officials who approve these drugs also benefit, because they get to perpetuate their jobs. And, not infrequently, some top regulators and the drug companies which they "regulate" actually work together quietly for their own benefits, *not* yours or mine.[1,2] As long as people are kept unhealthy and drug companies continue to develop toxic and sometimes useless drugs to ensure the future need of more drugs to counteract the problems caused by current ones, anyone involved in our sick-care system gets a piece of the money pie. That is, of course, except us, citizens who are *supposed* to be the ones benefitting. To put it bluntly, we are the victims. We are not only not healthier by taking these drugs, but are actually sicker, and getting even sicker every day because most of these drugs don't actually improve your health. They only temporarily relieve your existing symptoms, while at the same time produce others. The drug industry has been making so much money, and this money has infiltrated such a large portion of our sick-care system, that our elected officials and federal bureaucrats have no incentive to direct you away from drugs to other, healthier means of *genuine* health care. Insurance companies have also been so brain-washed by the drug industry and the medical establishment that they don't know better than to follow the drug-sickness-drug route. It has always been an uphill battle for honest and conscientious health care professionals and officials trying to buck the system by stressing preventive, genuine and alternative health care.

It often pains me to see friends and their families caught up in our country's sick-care system, totally trusting it, with serious adverse effects, both physically and financially. It affects me as well, because my insurance premiums and tax dollars go to support the cost of unnecessary drugs and surgery. The result is that their children are constantly visiting the doctor, getting antibiotics (yes, it still happens!) for their colds, undergoing one surgical procedure or another, and taking all sorts of drugs to relieve allergies and minor ills. These are the people who will eventually be forced to wake up (hopefully not too late) to see that they will be better off staying away from unnecessary visits to doctors and drugs. Unfortunately, this often happens only after some medical disaster.

My wife and I have raised two healthy daughters in the same environment as that of our friends. Both are now grown. During those years, apart from their yearly (required for camps) and later bi- or tri-yearly medical checkups and semi-annual dental care, they had rarely taken prescription or over-the-counter drugs, probably no more than once every few years. And their most serious operation was oral surgery to remove wisdom teeth.. However, they had occasionally taken herbal remedies in the form of herbs or foods, especially for viral infections such as colds and flu and allergies, which our modern medicines are notoriously inadequate in treating.

Once, our younger daughter asked us why she had never gone to the hospital, as some of her friends had done so frequently. We told her that it was because she was healthy and the hospital is a sick place to avoid. Nevertheless, when she later did volunteer work at a local hospital, we encouraged her because (despite our strong feelings about drugs) we believe modern medicine does have its place in our society. When they switched physicians from a pediatrician to a general practitioner and a gynecologist, their medical file was so thin that it prompted a nurse to remark that a month's record of many patients was thicker than those of our daughters' which had been accumulated over a 16-year period. Of course, it might be that we are just lucky to be blessed with good health. But I doubt it. We simply take good care of ourselves by not abusing our bodies and minds with drugs, including alcohol and tobacco, and avoiding going to the doctor unnecessarily and taking any prescription drugs. Also, we are educated enough and have observed enough physicians practice that we have not been taken in by the familiar phrase "consult your doctor," as we have found *that* to be definitely more to the benefit of the doctor than to the patient. I personally believe *that* to be a scare tactic to keep patients under the control of conventional doctors and drug interests. Indeed, it is rare that a patient leaves a physician's office without a prescription of some sort. And many patients are so conditioned by modern medicine that they expect drugs to be doled out every visit.

If the drug industry and the medical establishment depended on me and my family for business, they would both be bankrupt in short order. Don't get me wrong. I am anti-drug, but not a fanatic. I have been educated as a pharmacist, among other training. I do believe modern drugs should play a role in our health care, but not a predominant role. And I do occasionally (once every few years) consult my physician who happens to be one of the new breed of competent and compassionate medical practitioners with an open mind. Often, our modern diseases or illnesses are the result of our current "sick-care" system. If we take care of our health, we may never get these diseases or illnesses, and thus need not take drugs. One of the best ways to stay healthy is to stay away from drugs, any kind of synthetic drugs — chemicals that have suddenly appeared on the human scene only recently, even the safest and best of which have no more than two or three generations of so-called "safe" use history.

• • •

In contrast to these situations, certain foods and herbs have been safely used for thousands of years to keep us healthy. These are the ones I want to share with you in this book. They are the ones I most often use for my family's, friends', and my own personal health care needs.

Foods are to be experienced, enjoyed. So are herbs, many of which are also foods. Too often, when people start looking into the herbal field, they get so immediately involved with the alleged benefits or toxicities of an herb that they are quite confused, depending on which books they read. Here is the fact: No food or herb is totally safe or toxic. It all depends on how it is used and especially how it is prepared, whether by itself or with other herbs in combination. Also, all herbs, even well-known spices with thousands of years of safe use, may contain one or more ingredients that are toxic (if used in sufficient quantities), courtesy of diligent chemists who have been using more and more sophisticated methods to find them, even if often in only minute quantities. Thus, sage contains sizable quantities of thujone, which can cause convulsions if used in large doses or for prolonged periods. This chemical (also present in absinthium) is banned by the U.S. Food and Drug Administration (FDA). Our bureaucrats at the FDA either don't know what they are doing or they know their job too well. I prefer to give them the benefit of the doubt by considering the latter option: They took the long history of safe use of sage into account when they banned thujone in absinthium, but not in sage.

Indeed, many scientists often take the minor results of herb research too literally. Whenever they discover a toxic ingredient in an herb, irrespective of the amount present, they declare the herb to be toxic. A lot of times, consciously or subconsciously, they aggrandize themselves by trying to make their minor finding much more important than it actually is. Other times herbs have gotten their bad name through sloppy research by researchers who don't know anything about herbs, and who should not be doing research on herbs without collaboration with others who are trained in the field. A typical example that has gotten worldwide press and which was extensively quoted for the past fourteen years both in scientific and lay publications is the so-called "ginseng abuse syndrome." Results of that study were based on "capsules sold as ginseng," which could contain anything, including gums, starches and even sawdust for that matter, as well as toxic modern drugs, sometimes added by unethical manufacturers to give herbs a boost. These results were actually published in one of the most respected American medical journals.[3] It really boggles the mind to think how such sloppy research could have ever gotten published. My theory is that certain segments of the medical and scientific community are so prejudiced against herbs or so indebted to the drug industry that they will accept anything negative regarding herbs. It is sad to see scientists who otherwise pride themselves as unbiased researchers blinded by prejudice and greed, and who stoop so low to accept such shoddy work.

At the other end of the spectrum are certain herbalists who think herbs can do no wrong: herbs cure cancer, multiple sclerosis, heart diseases, or anything that ails you. These are the people who give herbs a bad name in the eyes of the scientific community. Then there are those who are not even interested in the benefits or "evils" of herbs, but instead see such a tremendous market in them that they find it extremely profitable to deal in them. They are the ones who supply the nutritional supplements industry with highly adulterated (diluted) extracts (*e.g.*, aloe vera and ginseng) at prices that are often below the cost of the genuine raw materials. The result is a mess. The average consumer has no way of knowing which products contain bogus or low-quality ingredients. These shysters have been responsible for much of the bad reputation accorded herbal supplements. The whole situation is not helped by various trade groups which openly advocate reform and quality control, yet whose major members include some of the worst offenders.

• • •

In this book, I have tried to bring out various important aspects relating to herbs or herbal foods that we frequently encounter during our day-to-day living. They may provide insight and may be useful in helping you make choices regarding herb/food use. The following is a summary of the main points I would like to get across:

- Frequently, when authors or researchers say there is "no published evidence" on a particular herb or its components, they don't mean there is actually no such evidence anywhere in the world. What they really mean is that *they don't have access* to such published evidence. What they should have said is "no published evidence available to us." A lot of the data in this book is derived from widely known published information in Chinese journals, much of which is now summarized and available in English for the first time in the second edition of my *Encyclopedia of Common Natural Ingredients Used in Food, Drugs and Cosmetics* (LEUNG AND FOSTER).
- There are usually numerous medicinal uses for any herb. Sometimes these uses are well documented through centuries of use. Other times these uses are personal opinion or experience of an individual writer, with no prior documentation. In this book, I have tried to include only the former.
- When an herb is described in an herb book as being remedial for a specific condition, it does not necessarily mean that it is indeed good for that condition if used indiscriminately. It may only be helpful for that particular condition if used along with other herbs or in certain concentrations, or processed in specific ways. Unfortunately, most often these stipulations are not described, and there is no way to find out except by trial and error. This is one of the reasons that doing research

on the efficacy of herbs is so difficult.

- One should not be alarmed by results of chemical and pharmacological research which shows that an herb contains toxic ingredients in minor amounts, or that one of the many chemical compounds in the herb is toxic when tested alone on experimental animals. Invariably, these findings are not relevant to our everyday living, except they may help boost the status and ego of the researchers concerned.
- If you are one of those people with an inquisitive and often skeptical mind, be sure to look into both sides of the story. Don't just take the word of someone with fancy scientific titles, nor that of some herbal guru claiming a large number of followers. Keep in mind that each of us has a distinctly different constitution. Herbs seem to work by delicately interacting with our body and balancing it to restore it to optimal function. Each person is different from the next in his or her reaction to these herbs. If the effects of herbs were overwhelming, like some highly toxic herbs and most modern drugs, our body would respond quickly, but it would then be thrown *out* of balance instead of *being* balanced by their effects. We might temporarily feel relieved or better, but our body system is still out of whack and will need to be brought back to balance. This is the way in which most modern drugs work. They may relieve symptoms, but they then cause others that eventually need to be dealt with.
- Herbs seem to work in pretty much the same way as do vitamins and minerals. Some herbs are rich in these nutrients while others contain only minor amounts. However, they contain other nutrients that so far have not been officially recognized by

conventional science. These nutrients include flavonoids, anthocyanidins, lignans, polysaccharides, glycosides, triterpenoids, sterols and some uncommon trace minerals. Taking a wide variety of herbs/foods (including common fruits, vegetable, nuts and grains) will insure us of an adequate supply of these nonconventional nutrients. Increasing scientific evidence has shown that many of these have very important functions in our body. Some of these functions are at the cellular level and their effects can be far-reaching. Thus, various flavonoids and lignans exhibit strong antioxidant properties while numerous polysaccharides have beneficial effects on our immune system. A new term, *nutriceuticals*, has been coined recently to describe some of these nutrients.

In a developed country like ours, even though we still have starving citizens (which is a national shame), most of us are no longer experiencing malnutrition. We rarely suffer from vitamin or mineral deficiency. However, we may be suffering from deficiencies of another kind. With our modern lifestyles come stress, polluted environments, unhealthy foods and toxic additives, and the effects of toxic modern drugs. All of these help rob our body system of nutrients, damage body cells and our immune system and thus weaken our body defenses. No wonder most of us don't have optimal health. But there is hope! The time will eventually come when the conventional medical and scientific communities and the federal bureaucrats will be forced to recognize nonconventional nutrients, and thus will make more herbs/foods available to the general public. But that will take time.

In the meantime, let the ignorant and the

biased take their hard drugs and conventional nutrients exclusively and continue to be barely able to cope. You and I will partake of the newly found nutrients, keep healthy and enjoy life. After all, these nutrients may have new names, but they have been around in the form of herbs and foods for centuries and millennia, enriching our health. They are not something a chemist has recently synthesized, with no prior safe use history and for which we have no idea about what cumulative damage will have been done to our bodies thirty years from now.

- There is a long-standing tradition of combining herbs, especially with Chinese herbs, to bring out the best function in certain herbs and tone down the harshness in others present in the same formula. This combination art has been practiced and perfected for centuries. Each herb in the formula has its place and may no longer have the same functions as when it is used by itself. Thus a toxic herb in a formula often is rendered harmless by others while the strength of an active herb is increased. One of the favorite lines of denigration used by conventional doctors and drug industry people relating to herbs and herbal formulas is, "Have they been clinically tested?" The answer is "Yes and no." If the question implies testing on animals and then human subjects over a period of less than a generation, the answer is "No." But if testing means actual use in humans through trial and error over a period of centuries and even millennia with safety and efficacy, the answer is a resounding "Yes." The ironic thing is that modern drug treatment has found out about the benefits of combinations and has started to use them. The question for the doctors and drug people with a closed mind should more appropriately be, "Are there financial incentives for me in these herbal formulas?"

- No food or herb is completely safe. There is always someone who is allergic to a particular herb or food. We have learned from experience what we can and cannot eat and to avoid or at least partake of less of those foods that make us uncomfortable. The same holds true with herbs that you have not used before. Be alert to any adverse reactions. If they occur, take less of the herb or stop taking it altogether if necessary. I am just being extra cautious. The fact is that herbs are probably one of the safest substances on earth to take. Consider this: Of all the complaints reported to the FDA in 1988 regarding side effects of food additives, 80% were due to Nutrasweet® (brand of aspartame), 15% were the result of sulfites, while the remaining were distributed among various categories. Herbs probably accounted for less than 1%.[4] So, chances are that you would more likely become ill by drinking diet soda than by taking an exotic herb.
- You should be aware that our FDA does not always act on your behalf, or does its best to protect your health. On the contrary; depending on who happens to be its politically appointed head, it sometimes makes decisions beneficial to its secret clients and detrimental to us. Thus, it was recently revealed that top officials who were involved in the approval of the genetically engineered drug rBGH (recombinant bovine growth hormone) which artificially stimulates cows to produce more milk, had close ties to the company that produces this drug.[1] This drug is now used by some large dairies to increase milk production by

up to 20%, and to thereby reap significantly greater profits.

There is nothing intrinsically wrong with this, with two exceptions. One, rBGH-treated cows are more prone to develop mastitis, requiring the increased use of antibiotics. These antibiotics could end up in our milk supply. Two, these high FDA officials actually approved the use of this new genetically engineered drug *without even requiring the milk producers to label the milk* as having been produced using rBGH. Consequently, we as consumers have no way of knowing which milk is produced using this drug, and which is not. Furthermore, smaller and/or more conscientious dairies whose milk is *not* produced using this hormone *cannot* even label their milk as *rBGH-free*, to give us a choice. Why? Because they are being sued by the former employers/clients of these FDA officials. The lawyers of the rBGH manufacturers rely heavily on the FDA-approved guidelines signed by one of its top officials, who incidentally has also been very biased against herbs. Surprise! Surprise!

• • •

It is no secret among academic and industrial experts that our FDA does not have personnel who are knowledgeable about herbs. Yet, this agency acts like a typical big bully (usually picking on little guys because it does not have the guts to pick on the big ones), trying to control and regulate herbs. This situation is analogous to having plumbers trying to do electrical work and to control and regulate electricians. Both specialties are essential to the construction and upkeep of your house. But would you tolerate this unprofessional conduct? Of course not! Unless you don't care about your house, that is. What we need instead is a separate body of knowledgeable herb experts to regulate herbs, not a group of biased and, at best, amateurish bureaucrats.

I am glad that our Congress has finally passed a bill titled *The Dietary Supplement Health and Education Act of 1994* which essentially removes herbs and vitamins from the realm of food additives and drugs, and out of the hands of the FDA. This is definitely a step in the right direction. Our nation may eventually be a healthy one yet!

In this book, the herbs and foods are listed in alphabetical order. **Properties** and **Most Common Traditional Uses** listed for each item are based on reliable sources that include classical and authoritative works, Some common uses that are of recent origin but with no traditional written records are also listed under **Other Advocated Uses** primarily to inform the reader that such uses exist and are worth noting. However, these uses may not have a long history. Also, under **Modern/Recent Uses** are described results of clinical uses that have been described in modern herbal and medical journals, which are mainly of Chinese origin. In describing Chinese traditional properties and uses, some organ terms are capitalized (*e.g.*, "nourishes Kidney and Liver," "Spleen-invigorating," etc.) to differentiate them from modern anatomical terms. Although the two have some common features, they are not equivalent. Thus, for instance, "Kidney" in Chinese medicine not only involves urinary functions, but sexual functions as well.

• • •

Note: The traditional and advocated food and herb uses reported in this book are not meant to be considered as prescribing medication. Rather, they are reported here for informational purposes only. Before using any herbal food that is not part of your regular diet, consult a knowledgeable health care professional or use caution as you would before starting any new regimen.

LIST OF HERBS AND FOODS

Alfalfa
Aloe Vera
Angelica
Astragalus
Baizhu
Bee Pollen
Cangzhu
Capsicum
Celery Seed
Cherokee Rosehip
Chicory
Chrysanthemum
Codonopsis
Dandelion
Danggui
Eleuthero
Fenugreek
Foti, Raw and Cured
Forsythia
Ganoderma
Garlic
German Chamomile
Giant Knotweed
Ginger
Ginseng, Asian and American
Gotu-kola
Hawthorn, Western and Chinese
Honeysuckle
Job's Tears
Jujube, Common
Juniper
Kudzu
Licorice
Ligustrum
Luffa
Lycium
Magnolia
Mume
Mung bean
Passion flower
Peony, Red and White
Poria
Purslane, Common
Red Sage
Rehmannia, Raw and Cured
Royal Jelly
Safflower
Sarsaparilla
Saw Palmetto
Schisandra
Sesame
Sour Jujube Kernel
Thyme
Turmeric
Watercress

ALFALFA (Syn. LUCERNE)

Plant Source: *Medicago sativa* L. (Family Leguminosae)
Part Used: Leaves and flowering tops
Properties: Appetizer, diuretic, tonic
Most Common Traditional Uses: To promote appetite and weight gain, to stop bleeding, to treat bladder stones and fluid retention
Other Advocated Uses: Arthritis, diabetes, peptic ulcer, alcoholism, to prevent absorption of cholesterol

Alfalfa is rich in nutrients, including proteins, antioxidant flavonoids, vitamins (A, B1, B6, B12, C, E and K), amino acids, minerals, sterols and fibers; it also contains saponin glycosides and coumarins. It is one of the commercial sources for chlorophyll production and is also a source for leaf protein production. Its extracts are used as flavor ingredients in many processed foods.

The popularity of alfalfa is quite recent, perhaps only a couple of decades. Although much chemical and pharmacological research has been performed on alfalfa, there is still no clear-cut evidence to support the benefits of alfalfa's advocated medicinal uses in humans. In addition, there is preliminary evidence that ingestion of large quantities of alfalfa (especially seeds or sprouts) may produce blood abnormalities and reactivate systemic lupus erythematosus in persons in whom this condition has been clinically inactive. Nevertheless, alfalfa does contain a wide variety of nutrients (both conventional and non-conventional) and ingestion of its leaves and sprouts in moderation can be quite nutritious. One thing to bear in mind is that nothing is absolutely safe, especially if done in excess. Also, it is *your* body, you know it the best. Continue to listen to it.

References: FOSTER AND DUKE; JIANGSU; LEUNG; LEUNG AND FOSTER; RICHARDSON; TYLER

ALOE VERA

Plant Source: *Aloe barbadensis* Miller (Family Liliaceae)
Part Used: Leaf gel
Properties: Healing, pain-relieving, emollient, soothing, antiinflammatory
Most Common Traditional Uses: *Internal*—General tonic, cleanser, detoxifier. *External* — Minor burns, sunburn, skin irritations, insect bites, minor cuts, scratches and wounds.
Other Advocated Uses: Too numerous to list

The external healing and pain-relieving properties of fresh aloe vera gel have been well established. The polysaccharides are believed to be the active principles. However, its other properties, especially internal, are still open to debate.

The internal uses of aloe gel appear to be only of recent origin, and lack long documented use history. Despite the controversy, aloe vera drinks (also called juices) have been consumed in tremendous quantities by the public for dozens of conditions, or for "whatever ails you." And there is no lack of testimonials to aloe vera's marvelous benefits. However, aloe vera is probably the most adulterated product on the world market, because most of the aloe drinks sold to consumers contain only a fraction of the claimed content of aloe vera gel. One fairly widely advertised "award-winning" brand claims to have no taste, contains no preservatives and keeps for years without spoiling; it actually tastes like water and looks like water, and probably *is* water!

Aloe vera is probably also the plant product that has produced the most millionaires in the United States, thanks to its name recognition and to the lack of testing methods to determine its quality. Greedy suppliers, brokers and manufacturers frequently stretch one gallon or one pound of genuine aloe vera gel liquid or powder to literally tens or hundreds of gallons or pounds of finished aloe drink, reaping outrageous profits. The taste of the aloe juice or drink you experience is mostly due to citric acid and preservatives. Genuine, fresh aloe gel tastes bland and slimy.

Aloe vera cosmetics are no better, because most of the time aloe vera gel is there just for a "label claim." This means that the product manufacturer merely puts in a minimum quantity of aloe so that its presence can be indicated on the label to entice you to buy it. The amount present is often so small that it imparts no benefit to the product (or consumer) whatsoever. You might have to try different brands until you find the right one that may contain enough aloe gel to do something for you.

Aloe vera gel normally contains no laxative ingredients (anthraglycosides). These laxative compounds are only present in special cells immediately beneath the skin of the leaf. After the leaf is cut crosswise, the yellow bitter latex containing these compounds drains out of the leaf. When this latex is dried, a dark resinous mass is produced which is commonly called simply "aloe." This aloe is a drug; it is used in many laxative preparations. A milder form of laxative is also produced from the aloe vera plant by splitting the whole leaf, drying it and then milling it to a powder. Since this product contains considerably lower amounts of anthraglycosides, and high concentrations of the gel, its laxative action is considered much less harsh than the concentrated aloe latex.

References: Leung; Leung and Foster; Lust; Ody; Tyler

ANGELICA

Plant Source: *Angelica archangelica* L. and other related *Angelica* spp. (Family Apiaceae)
Part Used: Root
Properties: Tonic, appetizer, carminative, expectorant, stimulant, stomachic, diuretic, diaphoretic, emmenagogic
Most Common Traditional Uses: Bronchial ailments, colds, coughs, stomach troubles, indigestion, flatulence, nervous conditions, insomnia, menstrual difficulties (cramps, pain, irregular menses, etc.), arthritis

In addition to a volatile oil, plant acids, sterols, flavonoids and other common constituents (starch, sugars, resin, etc.), angelica contains large amounts of coumarins, some of which (*e.g.*, bergapten and xanthotoxin) have strong phototoxic properties. Individuals who are sensitive to these compounds should exercise caution in handling angelica, as dermatitis may result if their skin comes in contact with these compounds and is then exposed to the sun.

Unlike the Chinese angelica (*danggui*), Western angelica does not have the long rich history and record of extensive use. However, angelica extracts are now used as a flavor ingredient in many types of foods, especially alcoholic beverages such as bitters, liqueurs, gin and vermouth.

References: Leung and Foster; Lust; Tyler

ASTRAGALUS (Syn. *Huangqi*)

Plant Source: *Astragalus membranaceus* (Fisch.) Bge. and other *Astragalus* spp. (Family Leguminosae)

Part Used: Root (raw and cured)

Properties: *Qi* (energy) tonic, healing, antiviral, antiinflammatory, antioxidant, immunomodulating, diuretic

Most Common Traditional Uses: *Raw root*—Spontaneous/night sweating, edema, painful joints, chronic sores/abscesses, nonhealing wounds and ulcers. *Cured root* — General weakness, fatigue, lack of appetite, diarrhea due to Spleen deficiency, rectal prolapse, uterine bleeding.

Modern/Recent Uses: Colds and flu, diabetes, stomach ulcer, neurodermatitis, AIDS

Documented use of astragalus root in China dates back at least two thousand years. It is one of the major *qi* (energy) tonics, being used in countless formulas as well as in various soup mixes. Although the raw and cured roots are distinctly different entities, some of their uses often overlap. Most of the above listed properties and uses have a documented scientific basis, some more extensive than others.

The chemistry and pharmacology of astragalus have been extensively studied, mainly by Chinese, Japanese and European researchers. It contains many types of chemical components. The ones found to be pharmacologically active so far include polysaccharides, triterpene glycosides, and flavonoids, none of which alone account for the overall properties of astragalus. Other pharmacological effects not listed above include hypotensive, vasodilating, improvement of learning and memory, liver protectant, and increase in stamina.

Astragalus, in combination with other traditional Chinese herbs (*e.g.*, licorice), is now widely used for its beneficial immunologic effects, especially in AIDS treatment by alternative health care physicians.

Astragalus is an herbal food with over two thousand years of safe use history. It contains a wide variety of both conventional (amino acids, minerals, etc.) and non-conventional (flavonoids, polysaccharides, triterpene glycosides, sterols, etc.) nutrients. It can serve as a source for both types of nutrients to help our body cope with the hardships of our modern lifestyle.

References: JIANGSU; LEUNG AND FOSTER; WANG 1; WANG 2

BAIZHU (Syn. Atractylodes)

Plant Source: *Atractylodes macrocephala* Koidz. (Family Asteraceae)

Part Used: Dried rhizome

Properties: *Qi* tonic, diuretic, invigorates Spleen, calms fetus

Most Common Traditional Uses: Indigestion, flatulence, diarrhea, fluid retention, spontaneous perspiration, restless fetus (excessive fetal movement)

Modern/Recent Uses: Constipation, leukopenia (low leukocyte count), toxic side effects of chemotherapy and radiotherapy

Baizhu is often simply called "atractylodes," but the latter term can also apply to *cangzhu*, a related but distinctly different herb. Hence *baizhu* products manufactured in America may in fact contain the wrong atractylodes. This is not surprising, as only in recent years have Chinese herbs become popular here, and many manufacturers and herbalists are still not knowledgeable about them. They tend to treat them as Western herbs that are much simpler in their selection, collection and initial treatment. Thus, like fo-ti, you are at the mercy of the manufacturers, who are often in turn at the mercy of their suppliers.

Like astragalus and ginseng, *baizhu* is one of the best known Chinese *qi* tonics. For over two thousand years, it has been safely used in soups, and its extracts in cakes and specialty rices, to maintain and improve health. Chemical studies have shown *baizhu* to contain up to 1.4% of a volatile oil (much less than that in *cangzhu* — up to 9.0%), sesquiterpene lactones, acetylenes, polysaccharides and others. Scientists have also found various pharmacologic effects in *baizhu* extracts and in one or more of *baizhu*'s chemical components. These effects include antiinflammatory, immunopotentiating, improving stamina, diuretic, hypoglycemic, liver protectant, anticoagulant and antitumor. Again, as with most modern studies on herbal tonics, none of their biological effects alone can account for *baizhu*'s traditional tonic properties. Nevertheless, when considered together, they do seem to show some scientific justification for *baizhu*'s traditional use to benefit our body when we are not in good health.

In recent years, *baizhu* has been effectively used in China in cancer chemotherapy and radiotherapy along with other tonic herbs (astragalus, licorice, etc.) to counteract the toxic side effects of these harsh treatments.

Baizhu is also used in skin care cosmetics for treating dark spots and wrinkles on the face and hands.

REFERENCES: CHP; JIANGSU; LEUNG AND FOSTER; PENG; WANG 1; WANG 2

BEE POLLEN

Plant Source: Variable, including buckwheat (*Fagopyrum esculentum* Moench), rape (*Brassica campestris* L.), pine (*Pinus* spp.) and *Typha* spp.
Part Used: Microspores (pollen) of male reproductive elements collected by bees
Properties: Nutrient, diuretic, hemostatic, breaks up stasis, astringent
Most Common Traditional Uses: Bleeding (nosebleed, vomiting blood, coughing blood, metrorrhagia, bloody diarrhea, traumatic injuries, etc.), amenorrhea, dysmenorrhea, abdominal pain, painful urination, mouth sores, eczema, alcohol intoxication, rheumatism
Modern/Recent Uses: Constipation

Much of the pollen used in the United States comes from China and Spain. Its sources are very different, hence its chemical composition reflects this. But in general it is very rich in nutrients, containing up to about 28% protein, 14.6 to 22.9% amino acids, 1 to 20% lipids, up to 44% carbohydrates, 2 to 2.5% flavonoids and 3.6 to 5.9% vitamin C. It also contains sterols, alkanes, triterpenes, etc.

Bee pollen can cause allergic reactions in some individuals. However, no serious toxic side effects due to its ingestion have been reported; otherwise, the news would have appeared on prime time television or on the front page of newspapers.

References: JIANGSU; LEUNG AND FOSTER; TYLER

CANGZHU (Syn. Atractylodes)

Plant Source: *Atractylodes lancea* (Thunb.) DC. [Southern *cangzhu*] and *A. chinensis* Koidz. ex Kitam. [Northern *cangzhu*] (Family Asteraceae)

Part Used: Dried rhizome

Properties: Invigorates Spleen, alleviates depression, antiarthritic, antirheumatic, disperses cold, improves vision, diuretic

Most Common Traditional Uses: Abdominal distension, diarrhea, lack of appetite, indigestion, edema, tiredness, sleepiness, rheumatism, arthritic pain, common cold, eczema, night blindness, warts

Modern/Recent Uses: Sterilization of operating rooms

Cangzhu contains up to 9.0% of a volatile oil and is much more aromatic than *baizhu* (the other atractylodes). The two were considered the same two thousand years ago and were simply known as *zhu* and grouped under the superior category of herbs in the Shennong Herbal (circa 200 B.C. — 100 A.D.) where other well-known tonics such as ginseng and astragalus were also grouped. However, as Chinese herbal medicine continued to develop, the two were found to have distinctly different properties, and were first recorded as separate herbs around 600 A.D. Since that time, although the two have some common properties and uses, *baizhu* is considered as a tonic and is commonly used as such, while *cangzhu* is not.

A traditional practice during an epidemic in China was to burn *cangzhu* to drive off the "evil" that was believed to cause the epidemic. The term "evil" or "evil wind," so commonly used in traditional Chinese medicine to describe one of the causes of illnesses, can often be correlated to "pathogens" in modern medicine. Having been trained in modern sciences and pharmacy, I used to be very skeptical about certain aspects of traditional Chinese medicine, even though I was brought up with it. It was not until after I had been seriously involved in it for a number of years, applying my scientific knowledge to analyze it with an open mind, that I find traditional Chinese medicine very logical, despite its often mysterious terminology. In my opinion, traditional Chinese medicine is also superior to modern medicine in many aspects of our health care, especially in viral infections such as colds and flus and in degenerative diseases, such as arthritis and rheumatism, as well as in keeping us healthy in the first place. Of course when you are really ill, almost beyond rescue, modern medicine may keep you alive with its modern technology while traditional Chinese medicine may not help you.

In recent years, the practice of burning *cangzhu* to drive off "evil" has been adopted in some local Chinese hospitals for the routine sterilization of operating rooms. The fumes from burning *cangzhu* are lethal to bacteria, viruses and fungi but are harmless to mosquitoes and insects as well as to humans and experimental animals; they are also non-irritating to humans and animals. However, the decoction and extracts of *cangzhu* do not have disinfectant effects.

REFERENCES: CHP; JIANGSU; LEUNG AND FOSTER; WANG 1

CAPSICUM (Syn. Red pepper, cayenne pepper, chili pepper, hot pepper)

Plant Source: *Capsicum frutescens* L., *C. annuum* L. and their hybrids and varieties (Family Solanaceae).

Part Used: Fruit

Properties: Rubefacient, stomachic, appetizer, carminative, circulatory stimulant, gastrointestinal stimulant, general tonic, antiinflammatory, analgesic

Most Common Traditional Uses: *Internal* — Digestive aid, flatulence, colic, cramps, diarrhea, toothache. *External* — Counter-irritant in arthritis and rheumatism, chilblain, frostbite, sprains, hematomas, poisonous snake bite.

Capsicum is rich in vitamins (A, C, β-carotene, etc.) and other nutrients. It is a favorite of Western herbalists who frequently use it in herbal formulas as a catalyst to enhance the effects of other herbs.

The major active constituent in capsicum is capsaicin, which has pain-relieving and antiinflammatory activities. It is also very irritating to mucous membranes and will cause intense pain when inadvertently rubbed into the eyes.

The traditional use of capsicum in treating arthritis and rheumatism now has a scientific basis in capsaicin, which is presently used in numerous external pain-relieving balms. The major drawback to these otherwise highly effective remedies is that extreme caution needs to be exercised in order to avoid accidental contact with mucous membranes, especially in and around the eyes.

References: Leung; Leung and Foster; Lust; Ody; Tyler

CELERY SEED (Syn. CELERY FRUIT)

Plant Source: *Apium graveolens* L. (Family Apiaceae)
Part Used: Fruit
Properties: Diuretic, digestive stimulant, nervine, muscle relaxant, emmenagogue, uterine stimulant
Most Common Traditional Uses: Rheumatism, arthritis, gout, bronchitis, nervousness

Celery seed contains numerous types of chemical components, including coumarin glycosides, flavonoids, phthalides, and plant acids. There is some scientific evidence to support its sedative and muscle-relaxant properties, with the phthalides being the active principles. The seed also has antioxidant effects.

Other parts of the celery plant have been reported to have hypotensive (juice and extract of stem) and antiinflammatory (water extract of stem) activities.

References: JIANGSU; LEUNG AND FOSTER; LUST; ODY; UPHOF

CHEROKEE ROSEHIP (Syn. CHINESE ROSEHIP; *JINYINGZI*)

Plant Source: *Rosa laevigata* Michx. (Family Rosaceae)
Part Used: Ripe fruit
Properties: Male tonic, antidiarrheal, antidiuretic, digestive aid, anti-atherosclerotic, antilipemic, antiviral, antimutagenic
Most Common Traditional Uses: Male sexual inadequacies (*e.g.* nocturnal emission, spermatorrhea, neurasthenia), female problems (*e.g.* leukorrhea, uterine bleeding), night sweating, excessive urination, bed wetting, chronic diarrhea, enteritis, chronic cough, high blood pressure

With its earliest written record dating back fifteen hundred years, Chinese rosehip is considered one of the most important Chinese health tonics. It is highly valued by the Chinese as both a food and a medicine. It is rich in both conventional and non-conventional nutrients, including especially vitamin C (~1.5%), saponin glycosides (~17%), flavonoids, carotenoids, leucoanthocyanidins, catechins, and plant acids, many of which have strong antioxidant properties.

Although all of the above uses have been well documented in traditional Chinese medical records, only its use in diarrhea and enteritis appears to be supported by modern scientific findings. Nevertheless, Chinese rosehip continues to be frequently used as a general and male tonic in countless preparations as well as in certain soup mixes for maintaining good health. Considering the abundance of such a variety of nutrients, I would not be surprised if this particular rosehip does indeed work, but in a manner we still don't understand.

References: JIANGSU; LEUNG AND FOSTER; LU AND LI; WANG 2

CHICORY

Plant Source: *Cichorium intybus* L. (Family Asteraceae)
Part Used: Root
Properties: Tonic, digestive aid, appetizer, cholagogue, diuretic, cardiotonic, mild laxative, antibacterial
Most Common Traditional Uses: Digestive problems, lack of appetite, liver and gallbladder ailments (*e.g.* gallstone, hepatitis, jaundice), spleen problems

Chicory root contains large amounts of inulin (up to 58% in fresh cultivated root), bitter principles (lactucin, intybin), coumarin glycosides, triterpenes, choline, and others. Inulin is made up of mostly fructose; although not digested by humans, it can serve as a potential source of commercial fructose after hydrolysis.

With its rich aroma and bitter taste, roasted chicory root is frequently mixed with coffee to enhance flavor and to reduce caffeine content. This practice is especially common in Europe.

References: JIANGSU; LEUNG AND FOSTER; LUST; RICHARDSON

CHRYSANTHEMUM (Syn. *Juhua*)

Plant Source: *Chrysanthemum indicum* L. (wild chrysanthemum) and *C. morifolium* Ramat. (florists' chrysanthemum) (Family Asteraceae)

Part Used: Flowerheads

Properties: Detoxicant, fever reducing, vision improving, antiinflammatory, antimicrobial (antibacterial, antifungal, antiviral), hypotensive

Most Common Traditional Uses: Common cold, flu, fever, headache, dizziness, redness of eyes, excessive tearing, skin sores, boils, abscesses, eczema

Modern/Recent Uses: High blood pressure, insomnia, angina pectoris, hepatitis

Although practically no Western scientific research, other than limited chemical studies, has been done on chrysanthemum, the ability of this herb to fight inflammations (*e.g.*, conjunctivitis), skin diseases and symptoms of hypertension has been well known in China for centuries. There is now scientific evidence to support its traditional use as a detoxicant (modern correlation: antibacterial, antiviral, antiinflammatory) to treat the above conditions.

Chrysanthemum is normally used as a tea. In recent years, it has become quite popular in Chinese restaurants in Hong Kong, where it is blended with *pu er cha* (a popular tea noted for its beneficial effects on digestion). This tea blend is now available in some Cantonese restaurants in major Chinatowns in North America.

Chrysanthemum flowers contain flavonoids, amino acids, and other nutrients (vitamin B1, adenine, choline, etc.) as well as a volatile oil. However, it may also contain sulfites. This is a result of traditional processing in which the fresh flowerheads are first fumigated with burning sulfur before drying in order to prevent mold growth and insect infestation. Those of you who are allergic to sulfites should be aware of this and drink chrysanthemum tea with caution. Chances are nothing will happen, as other ingredients in this "detoxifying" herb may neutralize the toxic effects of sulfites. But one can't be too cautious when it comes to trying something new.

Due to its detoxicant and antiinflammatory properties, chrysanthemum flower extracts are now used in cosmetics (creams, lotions, etc.).

References: CHEUNG AND LI; CHP; JIANGSU; LEUNG; WANG 2

CODONOPSIS (Syn. *Dangshen*)

Plant Source: *Codonopsis pilosula* (Franch.) Nannf. and other *Codonopsis* spp. (Family Campanulaceae)
Part Used: Root
Properties: *Qi* (energy) tonic, central stimulant, radioprotective, antistress, immunomodulating, hypotensive
Most Common Traditional Uses: General weakness, tiredness, lack of appetite, chronic diarrhea, asthma, cough, palpitations, shortness of breath, thirst, fever, diabetes
Modern/Recent Uses: High blood pressure, chronic anemia, leukemia

Considered as the poor man's ginseng, codonopsis is frequently used as a ginseng substitute to treat many of the same conditions as ginseng. Its documented use dates back only about three hundred years, but it has since become a highly valued *qi* tonic of status equal to that of some ancient ones (such as astragalus, ginseng and jujube). It is frequently used in combination with other herbs or in soup mixes to treat conditions due to Spleen and blood deficiencies as well as damaged *qi*. It is often used in "energy" formulas for its central stimulant effect as well as in formulas for boosting one's immune system.

Codonopsis contains large amounts of polysaccharides and sugars (inulin, starch, glucose, sucrose, fructose, etc.), saponins (tangshenosides, but no ginsenosides), amino acids, alkaloids, triterpenes, sterols, volatile oil, oroxylin A, and trace minerals, among others.

Its extracts have been shown to increase blood sugar levels in animals, yet codonopsis is traditionally used to treat diabetes. This appears to be another case of contradiction in herbal research. Nevertheless, many of the other traditional uses have been corroborated by Western Science.

References: CHP; JIANGSU; LEUNG AND FOSTER; WANG 1; WANG 2

DANDELION

Plant Source: *Taraxacum officinale* Wiggers, *T. mongolicum* Hand.-Mazz. and other *Taraxacum* spp. (Family Asteraceae)

Part Used: Root and leaves

Properties: Tonic, detoxifier, fever reducer, mild laxative, diuretic, choleretic, antiinflammatory, antimicrobial (antibacterial, antifungal, antiviral), hypoglycemic

Most Common Traditional Uses: Liver and spleen problems (jaundice, gallstones), rheumatism, stiff joints, gout, skin problems (eczema, sores, etc.), bruises, breast problems (inflammation, lumps, lack of milk flow, etc.), constipation, lack of urine flow

Modern/Recent Uses: Bacterial and viral infections (upper respiratory tract, urinary tract, chronic bronchitis, mumps, pneumonia, hepatitis, etc.), lack of appetite, indigestion, flatulence

Yes, this is the weed most American home owners consider a pest. However, different parts of the plant have been used since ancient times by different cultures as medicines. Roasted root is used as coffee substitute or flavor enhancer; flowers are made into wine, and fresh leaves are eaten raw as salad or cooked as vegetables.

The Chinese use the whole plant (root and all) extensively to treat "hot and toxic" conditions which in modern terms are correlated broadly with bacterial and viral infections which produce fever and swelling, including skin diseases such as sores, carbuncles and furuncles. There is substantial scientific evidence to support its traditional uses as a detoxicant (antibacterial, antiviral, antiinflammatory, antitumor) and digestive tonic.

Dandelion is very closely related to chicory; its root also contains high concentrations of inulin (see chicory). In addition, the root is rich in triterpenes, bitter principles (sesquiterpene lactones), sterols, phenolic acids and other nutrients.

Dandelion greens are very rich in vitamins A, B, C and D and carotenoids. In fact, its vitamin A content is higher than that of carrots.

References: Jiangsu; Leung; Leung and Foster; Lust; Wang 2

DANGGUI (Syn. CHINESE ANGELICA, *DONG QUAI, TANG KUEI*)

Plant Source: *Angelica sinensis* (Oliv.) Diels.(Family Apiaceae)

Part Used: Root

Properties: Blood tonic (purifies blood, promotes blood formation and circulation, regulates menstrual flow), moisturizes and lubricates the intestines

Most Common Traditional Uses: Menstrual disorders (irregular menses, metrorrhagia, amenorrhea, cramps, pain, etc.), anemia, weakness due to loss of blood, insomnia, headache, constipation, boils and ulcers, traumatic injuries

Modern/Recent Uses: High blood pressure, rheumatism, arthritic pain, muscle pain, neuralgia, shingles

Chinese angelica is known in English under numerous names, including *danggui, dong quai, tang kwei, tang kuei, dang qui,* etc. Only two of these are the officially "correct" names, *danggui* and *tang kuei.* The former is based on the official Chinese *pinyin* transliteration system and is closest to the actual pronunciation in Chinese (Mandarin). The latter, *tang kuei,* is based on the older Wade-Giles transliteration system which is less accurate and is now only used in Taiwanese and other free-world publications which represent only a minor proportion of all Chinese publications.

With its first recorded use dating back two thousand years, *danggui* is perhaps the most widely used tonic in the world, especially among Chinese women. It is eaten in soups and popular dishes such as "*danggui* duck" and "*danggui* chicken." While growing up in a household of mostly women, I often ate these dishes. Although *danggui* is primarily for women, it can be consumed by men as well.

Since its recent introduction to the American health food market, *danggui* has increasingly gained popularity among American women for their menstrual problems. As it has a very strong and distinct odor, it is difficult for dishonest manufacturers and marketers to cut it too much with cheap and inert fillers. Consequently, unlike other expensive herbs (*e.g.*, ginseng and aloe vera), *danggui* products can be identified by their unique fragrance. As a general rule, the stronger the odor, the better the product (at least for now, or until the shysters find a cheap synthetic odor to pass off as *danggui*).

Like other tonics, *danggui* acts very subtly in our body. It would be extremely difficult to prove its effectiveness one way or the other by modern clinical trials. But with over two thousand years of safe and beneficial use, who needs them? The only people who want clinical trials are the drug industry and associated government bureaucrats who stand to lose big financially if American women don't need drugs to take care of problems associated with menstruation.

Incidentally, you may have heard something about the Canadian government requiring a cautionary pregnancy label for *danggui* products. I have no idea where they obtained the data on which they based their decision, but I suspect it was based on misinformation as well as prejudice against herbal products. First, in laboratory studies, *danggui* has been shown to have *both* stimulatory and inhibitory effects on the uterus and other smooth muscles of animals. That should tell you that one can't treat a tonic herb like *danggui* as if it were a single synthetic chemical. Second, there is no record in the traditional Chinese literature warning against its use in pregnancy. On the contrary, it is well known for its "fetus-calming" properties and is sometimes prescribed along with other herbs to prevent abortion and to treat other pregnancy-associated conditions. My personal opinion is that some bureaucrat had confused lovage with the real *danggui* because the former is also known in China as "European *danggui*."

Unlike *danggui*, lovage is not recommended for use during pregnancy.

References: CHP; JIANGSU; LEUNG AND FOSTER; LUST; WANG 1

ELEUTHERO (Syn. Siberian ginseng; *ciwujia*)

Plant Source: *Eleutherococcus senticosus* (Rupr. and Maxim.) Maxim. (Family Araliaceae)
Part Used: Dried root and rhizome
Properties: Tonic, stimulant, adaptogenic, strengthens tendons and bones, removes rheumatism, invigorates blood and breaks up blood stasis, diuretic
Most Common Traditional Uses: Rheumatism, arthritis, backache, edema, weakness of legs, impotence, traumatic injuries
Modern/Recent Uses: Stress, low resistance to diseases

Eleuthero, or *ciwujia*, is one of several *wujias* that have been used interchangeably for over two thousand years in China as a general tonic to treat various conditions. Although also called Siberian "ginseng" with tonic properties like ginseng and belonging to the same family, eleuthero contains active constituents that are quite different from those of ginseng. Thus, it does not contain the well-known saponin glycosides (called ginsenosides) which are the major active principles of ginseng. Instead, its active components (called eleutherosides) are glycosides of sterols, phenylpropanoids, coumarins, lignans and triterpenes. It also contains other nutrients such as vitamins (E, β-carotene, etc.) and polysaccharides, among others.

As typical in research on tonics, bits and pieces of scientific evidence have shown eleuthero to have broad biological effects, including hypoglycemic, antiinflammatory, diuretic, estrogenic, gonadotropic, antihypertensive, antioxidant, immunomodulating, antitumor, antiedema, stress-resistant, etc. Although some of the activities have been attributed to certain eleutherosides and polysaccharides in eleuthero, the fact remains we still don't know how and why eleuthero works. Instead of looking for a single chemical hoping it will give us the key to eleuthero's secrets, we should be evaluating the whole herb. The problem is that based on the current system of drug research support, no drug company or government agency would be interested in supporting work which is not on a single patentable chemical. Well-known herbs and formulas cannot be patented and without a patent, the financial supporter or its associates and friends cannot make big money.

References: CHP; Jiangsu; Leung and Foster

FENUGREEK

Plant Source: *Trigonella foenum-graecum* L. (Family Leguminosae)

Part Used: Ripe seed

Properties: Digestive, expectorant, fever-reducing, aphrodisiac, male tonic, pain-relieving, demulcent, emollient, promoting milk flow, uterine stimulant, hypoglycemic

Most Common Traditional Uses: Fever, sore throat, bronchitis, mouth ulcers, chapped lips, chronic cough, gout, neuralgia, sciatica, swollen glands, skin sores, furuncle, irritations, impotence, spermatorrhea, premature ejaculation, kidney ailments, beriberi, hernia, abdominal pain

Fenugreek has been used since ancient times as a medicine and food or spice in Egypt, India and the Middle East, but has been adopted by the Chinese for only about a thousand years. While the Chinese consider fenugreek as a warming herb, other cultures use it to treat fevers and other "hot" conditions (*e.g.* swollen glands, sore throat, skin sores, furuncle) that are normally treated in Chinese medicine with cooling herbs.

None of the scientific studies on fenugreek published so far appear to have any relevance to its traditional uses except, perhaps, its chemistry. Chemically, it is rich in steroid precursors (from which steroid drugs can be produced), flavonoids (many of which have strong antioxidant properties), mucilage (maybe the demulcent and emollient principle), protein and other nutrients (amino acids, vitamins A, B1 and C, etc.). These compounds may contribute to its traditional properties.

Also, a statement in an early 16th Century Chinese herbal advising pregnant women not to use fenugreek seems to have some scientific rationale, as it has been found to stimulate animal uteruses in the laboratory. But don't be prematurely alarmed! Fenugreek is a major ingredient of curry which has been safely used over centuries by billions of people, many of whom were no doubt pregnant. The key, as always, is the amount ingested. Again, let's not forget the word "moderation."

References: CHP; JIANGSU; LEUNG AND FOSTER; LUST; ODY; UPHOF

FO-TI, RAW and CURED (Syn. *He-shouwu, polygonum*)

Plant Source: *Polygonum multiflorum* Thunb. (Family Polygonaceae)

Part Used: Root tuber

Properties: *Raw Fo-ti* — Detoxicant, laxative, liver protectant, antioxidant, hypolipemic, antibacterial. *Cured Fo-ti* — Tonic (blood, Liver and Kidney), antioxidant, immunostimulant, anti-atherosclerotic, hypolipemic, antiviral, antibacterial.

Most Common Traditional Uses: *Raw Fo-ti* — Scrofula, sores, carbuncles, skin eruptions, pruritus, inflammations, constipation, hyperlipemia. *Cured Fo-ti* — Dizziness, tinnitus, insomnia, premature graying, hair loss, numbness of limbs, weak knee and back, soreness of knees and back, general weakness, hyperlipemia.

Raw and cured fo-ti are different both in preparation and in traditional properties and uses. Raw fo-ti is simply the cleaned and dried root tuber; while cured fo-ti has undergone a complicated prolonged cooking process with black soybean broth. Raw fo-ti is over fifty times more toxic than cured fo-ti and has strong laxative properties. In contrast, cured fo-ti is relatively nontoxic and has little or no laxative effects, as processing destroys most of the laxative ingredients but increases the immunostimulating components. As most American herbalists and manufacturers are not familiar with the intricacies of Chinese herbs, they often don't distinguish raw fo-ti from cured fo-ti. Hence, the much cheaper raw fo-ti is frequently used, no matter which is called for. I have personally come across the raw form being offered to major health food manufacturers as cured fo-ti. So watch out!

Cured fo-ti is regarded by the Chinese as one of the most important anti-aging herbs and is extensively used in tonic formulas. Modern scientific findings seem to support the rationale of many of its traditional uses.

References: CHP; JIANGSU; LEUNG AND FOSTER; TYLER; WANG 1; WANG 2

FORSYTHIA (Syn. *Lianqiao*)

Plant Source: *Forsythia suspensa* (Thunb.) Vahl. (Family Oleaceae).

Part Used: Ripe fruit with or without seeds

Properties: Disperses heat, removes swelling, breaks up nodules, detoxicant, antiviral, antibacterial, antipyretic, antiinflammatory, hypotensive, antioxidant, liver protectant

Most Common Traditional Uses: Colds and flus and associated symptoms, fevers, skin rashes, urination difficulties, inflammation of lymph nodes, infectious diseases (*e.g.*, erysipelas)

Modern/Recent Uses: Allergies

Forsythia fruit is one of the most common components in Chinese herbal formulas for treating the common cold, influenza and allergies (*e.g.*, hay fever). With continuous documentation of at least three thousand years, it is traditionally considered a detoxicant for treating so-called "toxic" and "hot" conditions. These conditions correlate with modern inflammatory and infectious diseases, including viral and bacterial infections, as well as allergies. The properties and uses of forsythia fruit now appear to have considerable scientific support.

In recent laboratory studies, Chinese scientists have found its decoction (water extract) and other extracts (*e.g.*, alcohol extract) to have antiviral, antibacterial, antiinflammatory, antipyretic, antiallergic and antioxidant activities *in vitro* and in experimental animals. Chemical studies have revealed various active constituents, including relatively large amounts of oleanolic acid (0.73 to 2.28%) and other triterpenes, phenols (*e.g.* forsythol), sterols and flavonoids. Although oleanolic acid has antiallergic and liver protectant and forsythol antibacterial activities, they cannot account for the varied biological effects and total traditional properties of forsythia fruit. Again, this is nothing new when it comes to scientific investigations of herbs using the typical single-chemical drug approach, where researchers are only looking for a one-to-one effect. In herbal medicine, there is no such thing. At best you are looking at a rare occasion where a single chemical of an herb is responsible for one or two of its specific properties, such as ephedrine from *mahuang (Ephedra* spp.), berberine from *huanglian* (*Coptis* spp.) and quinine from cinchona bark. However, these specific chemicals with specific effects don't account for the total traditional properties and uses of these herbs.

Like other scientists, I don't have a clear idea how forsythia fruit works in taking care of colds, flus and allergies. But based on personal experience with this and related herbs and after almost twenty years of intensive searching and accumulating traditional and modern Chinese herbal data, including a collection of most of the major Chinese herbals ever published and over sixty modern Chinese journals (quarterly, bimonthly and monthly) on traditional herbal medicine, I can tell you that traditional Chinese formulas for treating "toxic" and "hot" conditions are superior to modern cold, flu and allergy medicines. Some of these formulas have been safely used for hundreds of years.

While modern medicines only offer temporary relief of symptoms (often simultaneously causing toxic side effects), the traditional Chinese herbal formulas take care of the virus ("evil") as well as strengthen the body, with much less toxic side effects, if any at all. My family and friends have been using two to three of these formulas with considerable success. I would be very upset if I were forced to use modern drugs by some biased and self-serving bureaucrats; so would my family and friends.

Extracts of forsythia fruit are now also used in numerous types of cosmetic products, including hair care (*e.g.*, hair growth liniments and antidandruff shampoos), skin care (*e.g.*, acne cream) and foot care (*e.g.*, athlete's foot) products for their antimicrobial and traditional detoxifying properties.

REFERENCES: CHP; JIANGSU; LEUNG AND FOSTER; WANG 1

GANODERMA (Syn. *Reishi; lingzhi*)

Plant Source: *Ganoderma lucidum* (Leyss. ex Fr.) Karst. [red *lingzhi*] and *G. japonicum* (Fr.) Lloyd. [purple *lingzhi*] (Family Polyporaceae)

Part Used: Fruiting body (mushroom)

Properties: General tonic, benefits *qi* (energy), improves memory, benefits complexion, eases joint movement, strengthens tendons and bones, calms nerves

Most Common Traditional Uses: General weakness, cough, asthma, insomnia, indigestion

Modern/Recent Uses: Nightmares, neurasthenia, heart problems (coronary heart disease, arrhythmia, hyperlipemia, hypertension, etc.), lack of appetite, chronic hepatitis, mushroom poisoning, chronic bronchitis, leukocytopenia

Ganoderma is known as *lingzhi* in Chinese and *reishi* or *mannentake* in Japanese. It was the "elixir of life" sought by emperors and sages during most of China's long history, and has been glorified in Chinese literary classics, with a reputation as a tonic to prolong life matching that of ginseng.

Both ganodermas are widely distributed in China, especially along coastal provinces. *Ganoderma lucidum* is also found growing on hardwoods in North America. Until recent years, ganoderma was rather rare and was primarily reserved for the privileged classes. But since the successful cultivation of *G. lucidum,* it is now readily available both from the Far East as well as the United States and Canada.

During the past few decades, hundreds of scientific studies (especially chemical and pharmacological) on ganoderma have been published, mostly by Japanese and Chinese researchers. These scientists have found ganoderma to contain many types of biologically active chemical constituents, including sterols, triterpenes, polysaccharides, fatty acids, amino acids, peptides, adenosine, betaine, alkaloids and trace minerals (high in germanium), among others. Its pharmacological activities are very broad, including sedative, analgesic, anticonvulsive, hypertensive and hypotensive, anti-allergic, liver protectant, hypoglycemic, antitumor, anticoagulant, hypolipemic and hypercholesterolemic, anticholinergic, antioxidant, immunomodulating, smooth muscle relaxant, antitussive, antiasthmatic, vasodilative, diuretic, anabolic, antiinflammatory, anti-fatigue and antibacterial, etc. Even though these are isolated studies, the sheer quantity of bioactivity seems to give some justification of ganoderma's good reputation as a highly valued general tonic. Let's face it, there is no way one can subject a tonic like ganoderma (or ginseng) to so-called clinical trials (double-blind, randomized, etc.) and expect to obtain meaningful results.

As an observant reader, you would have noticed that ganoderma has both hypotensive and hypertensive as well as both hypolipemic and hypercholesteremic effects. These are opposite effects and the kind of research results that would drive some scientists nuts, especially those looking for one drug/one effect. Some biochemists and pharmacologists may try to explain these findings in fancy technical terms, with elaborate theories and mechanisms of action. But the fact is that they may not have the foggiest idea why ganoderma exhibits opposite effects. Me? I don't know either. But I would simply attribute all these effects to Mother Nature's work being superior to those of human endeavors; you just can't simply break it down to fit our limited scope of understanding.

References: JIANGSU; LEUNG AND FOSTER; WANG 2

GARLIC

Plant Source: *Allium sativum* L. (Family Liliaceae)
Part Used: Bulb
Properties: Cure-all, including anthelmintic, antispasmodic, carminative, cholagogue, digestive, diuretic, expectorant, febrifuge, aphrodisiac, hypotensive, antibacterial
Most Common Uses: Coughs, colds, chronic bronchitis, toothache, earache, dandruff, hypertension, arteriosclerosis, hysteria, rheumatism, gout, ulcers, diarrhea, dysentery, pulmonary tuberculosis, bloody urine, hepatitis, diphtheria, whooping cough, trachoma, hypersensitive dentin, vaginal trichomoniasis, scalp ringworm, typhoid, stomachache, headache, sinus congestion

If any herb qualifies as a cure-all, garlic is the one. There is probably as much hype as there is scientific validity to many of its uses. If you believe some of the "modern" findings about garlic's effectiveness, you will probably never eat garlic (raw or cooked) for health again! Instead, you would only opt for garlic pills specially coated to deliver it to the right area in your body.

Over a thousand scientific papers on garlic have appeared in recent years, yielding results showing garlic to have many pharmacologic activities. But again, as with any herb which has tonic or multiple functions, all these scientific findings don't amount to much in proving garlic's actions one way or the other. It is fine if you are interested in a particular chemical in garlic as a specific drug. You can isolate it and turn it into one. But don't try to connect it with garlic itself, because by now one should know garlic does not have one or two so-called active principles. Chances are the traditional value of garlic does not lie in one or two chemicals but rather in the total combination of different components working together.

Incidentally, for those who are interested in taking garlic preparations, the most common conditions for which garlic is indicated include arteriosclerosis, hyperlipemia, coronary artery disease, hypertension, and bacterial/fungul infections. Again, there is no guarantee that the particular brand you buy is effective

References: JIANGSU; LEUNG; LEUNG AND FOSTER; LUST; ODY; TYLER; WANG 1; WANG 2

GERMAN CHAMOMILE

Plant Source: *Matricaria recutita* L. (Family Asteraceae)
Part Used: Flowerheads
Properties: Antiinflammatory, pain relieving, calmative, antispasmodic, diaphoretic, carminative, tonic, anti-infective, wound-healing
Most Common Traditional Uses: Colic, indigestion, inflammation of the G.I. tract, peptic ulcers, insomnia, infantile convulsions, toothache, bleeding and swollen gums, sciatica, gout, lumbago, skin problems (bacterial infections, inflammations, etc.)

German chamomile contains a blue volatile oil, flavonoids, proazulenes, coumarins, amino acids, choline, etc. Chamazulene, β-bisabolol and en-yn-dicycloether in the volatile oil are some of the active principles responsible for chamomile's antiinflammatory, antimicrobial and antispasmodic properties. The medicinal use of chamomile is especially popular in Europe, though it is gaining popularity in America as well. It is normally used as a tea.

Another chamomile (*Anthemis nobilis* L.), also known as English or Roman chamomile, has basically the same properties and uses as German chamomile. However, English chamomile causes many more reported incidences of allergic reactions in humans than does German chamomile. Thus, between the years 1887 and 1982, 45 cases of adverse reactions were reported for English chamomile in contrast to 5 cases for German chamomile. These numbers are minuscule compared to the large numbers of toxic reactions reported to the FDA (80% of all complaints received in 1988) relating to the use of Nutrasweet (aspartame).[4]

References: LEUNG AND FOSTER; LUST; ODY; TYLER

GIANT KNOTWEED (Syn. *Huzhang*)

Plant Source: *Polygonum cuspidatum* Sieb. et Zucc. (Family Polygonaceae)
Part Used: Root and rhizome
Properties: Antiarthritic, antirheumatic, analgesic, detoxicant, antitussive, expectorant, antibacterial, antiviral, antioxidant
Most Common Traditional Uses: Painful joints, jaundice, menstrual difficulties, cough with excessive phlegm, skin sores and boils, traumatic injuries
Modern/Recent Uses: Burns, acute viral hepatitis, acute infections (*e.g.*, appendicitis)

Originally native to eastern Asia, giant knotweed has escaped in North America and is now a weed found throughout New England and neighboring states and in Canada. Young shoots are edible. Despite its abundance here in America, the rhizome and root are not collected or used, and *huzhang* comes primarily from China.

Although *huzhang* is botanically very closely related to fo-ti and buckwheat, their major uses differ considerably. Whereas fo-ti (especially the cured form) and buckwheat have a long history of use as a tonic or food, the use of *huzhang* is limited to specific disease treatments. In recent years, the Chinese have been using *huzhang* in the treatment of burns and acute viral hepatitis with considerable success. Modern scientific studies performed by Chinese and Japanese researchers have found that some of *huzhang*'s chemical components have antibacterial, antiviral, liver protectant and antioxidant effects.

The unique broad, traditional and modern properties of *huzhang*, which include detoxicant, antiburn, wound healing, astringent, antimicrobial and antioxidant, have been utilized in skin care cosmetics and environmental products. Its extracts are used in skin lotions, antifatigue, massage and cleansing creams as well as in an herbal disinfectant recently approved by the U.S. Environmental

Protection Agency (EPA).

References: CHP; JIANGSU; LEUNG AND FOSTER; RICHARDSON; WANG 1; WANG 2

GINGER

Plant Source: *Zingiber officinale* Roscoe (Family Zingiberaceae)

Part Used: Rhizome ("root")

Properties: Carminative, diaphoretic, appetite stimulant, antiemetic, antinausea, digestive aid, antiinflammatory, pain relieving, detoxifier, tonic

Most Common Traditional Uses: Common cold, sore throat, wheezing, cough, excessive phlegm, nasal congestion, nausea, vomiting, abdominal distension, stomachache, diarrhea, bleeding, adverse effects of drugs and foods (*e.g.*, seafood)

Modern/Recent Uses: Malaria, rheumatic pain, intestinal hernia, stomach and duodenal ulcers, dysentery, inflammation of the testes, drug poisoning, topically for nonhealing sores, hemorrhoids, burns, peeling skin and toothache

In addition to being a common spice, ginger has been used for thousands of years as a medicine by different cultures for the above conditions. In China, ginger is one of the most widely used herbs in formulas, and it is often used with black soybean, mung bean and/or licorice to treat food and chemical poisoning. In recent years, fresh ginger juice has found a new use in China in the treatment of burns.[5] Contrary to popular belief or misconception, ginger juice when applied to unopened burns does not sting, but rather offers immediate relief.

During the past several years, ginger has gained increasing popularity as a relief for motion sickness, especially after a series of clinical trials showing its effectiveness were reported. However, before all the current Western interest in this particular use, the Chinese had been using it for centuries. I remember as a boy my relatives from the country used to bring along preserved ginger to munch on when they came to visit us by bus or by boat. The Chinese learned about this property of ginger over centuries of practical experience and have been quietly benefiting from it all this time. Yet if our American bureaucrats had their way, they would tell us that we could not tell others about our experience. Instead, we would only be allowed to take drugs developed by their colleagues, the drug companies, paying exorbitant prices for them, not to mention experiencing the toxic side effects of these drugs!

References: CHP; Jiangsu; Leung; Leung and Foster; Lust; Ody; Tyler; Wang 1; Wang 2

GINSENG, ASIAN (Formerly ORIENTAL) and AMERICAN

Plant Source: *Panax ginseng* C.A. Mey. (Asian) and *Panax quinquefolius* (American) [Family Araliaceae]

Part Used: Dried root, raw or cured

Properties: *Asian Ginseng* — Warming, general tonic, stimulant, anti-stress, radioprotective, immunomodulating, sedative, hypotensive, hypoglycemic. *American Ginseng* — Cooling, thirst-quenching, febrifuge, tonic.

Most Common Traditional Uses: *Asian Ginseng* — General weakness, tiredness, mental and physical exhaustion (especially after a long illness), cold limbs, weak heart, insomnia, lack of appetite, impotence, rheumatism, etc. *American Ginseng* — Fever, summer heat (*e.g.* sunstroke), thirst.

Ginseng needs no introduction; few have not heard of it. It is in fact the best known Chinese herb in the world. Although it has many properties and uses, decades of scientific research and thousands of publications have not proven its capabilities one way or the other. Is it what it is alleged to be? We may never know. And science may never determine what it sets out to ascertain. A couple of well-known facts: Asian ginseng has been highly valued and used by billions of Chinese over at least two thousand years; and the Chinese are not a stupid people.

A distinction should be made between Asian and American ginseng. Asian ginseng is warming and is good for people who have recovered from a serious illness and need to regain their strength; it is used as a general tonic to strengthen the body's resistance. It should not be used by people with excessive *yang,* including a ruddy complexion and energetic constitution. On the other hand, American ginseng has cooling properties and is normally used to cool down fevers or summer heat. It is good for people with deficient *yin* or excessive *yang*.

If you are prone to cold hands and feet, lack of energy, or are generally not quite up to snuff, you should take Asian ginseng. But if you are usually the hyperactive type, often hot, and full of vigor, you should not take Asian ginseng but rather American ginseng. American ginseng root and Asian ginseng *leaf* are also used to treat hangovers.

The active components of ginseng (both Asian and American) are numerous, including ginseng saponins (ginsenosides and panaxosides) and polysaccharides. Together they are responsible for the total effects of ginseng. You may have heard about "standardized" ginseng products. This means that these products contain a measurable amount of ginsenosides, usually only one or two of several dozen of such compounds. It has been assumed by some Western scientists that ginsenosides are the only active principles in ginseng and since these chemicals can be measured, we can at least be sure that these products contain some active components, rather than inert diluents like starch and sugar. Nevertheless, unless these products contain ginsenosides from a total extract of ginseng (highly unlikely in the concentrated ginseng extracts), chances are the other active principles are not there. Hence, the best way to take ginseng is to buy the root from Chinatown herb shops and brew the tea yourself, because prepared ginseng products often don't tell you which ginseng they contain. Sometimes they may bear one specific plant name on the label, but the other plant may be actually the one used, as some manufacturers themselves don't know the difference between the two. To make ginseng tea, simply steep 1 to 2 level teaspoonfuls of the ground root or crushed leaf in a cup of boiling water for 5 to 10 minutes.

References: LEUNG; LEUNG AND FOSTER; TYLER; WANG 2

GOTU-KOLA

Plant Source: *Centella asiatica* (L.) Urban (Family Apiaceae)
Part Used: Leaves or whole herb
Properties: Wound-healing, detoxicant, antiinflammatory, diuretic, pain-relieving, antibacterial
Most Common Traditional Uses: Traumatic injuries, swellings, skin sores and boils, skin eruptions (*e.g.*, measles), sunstroke, fever, common cold
Modern/Recent Uses: Wounds, skin ulcers, burns, leprosy, scleroderma, traumatic pain, jaundice, hepatitis, poisoning (arsenic, mushroom, cassava, etc.), syphilis, mental problems

Gotu-kola is not to be confused with kola nuts (*Cola nitida*); the latter contain caffeine while the former doesn't.

Gotu-kola has been used by different cultures worldwide both as a medicine and as a food for centuries. The young plant is cooked or pickled and eaten as a vegetable in Southeast Asia. It has been used as a medicine for thousands of years in China and India and its use there has been documented for at least two thousand years.

The active principles of *gotu-kola* are currently attributed to triterpenoid saponin glycosides (wound-healing, antimicrobial, sedative, antiinflammatory, etc.) though other components present may also contribute to its total beneficial effects; they include steroids, fatty acids, flavonoids and other polyphenols.

Although *gotu-kola* is also advocated as an anti-aging herb and an aphrodisiac, so far there has been no credible evidence to correlate such effects.

The raw herb comes in highly variable qualities. Some are extremely dirty, with leaves mostly broken and containing large quantities of mud and dirt. Consequently, one should avoid the powdered herb unless it is from a reliable supplier, because it is a common industrial practice to use inferior quality materials to produce herb powders.

Reference: Cheung and Li; CHP; Jiangsu; Leung and Foster; Tyler

HAWTHORN, WESTERN and CHINESE

Plant Source: *Crataegus* spp. (Family Rosaceae) [WESTERN HAWTHORN (English and European) — *C. laevigata* (Poir) DC and *C. monogyna* Jacq.; CHINESE HAWTHORN (*shanzha*) — *C. pinnatifida* Bge. and *C. cuneata* Sieb. et Zucc.]

Part Used: Dried fruits; also leaves and flowering tops (Western hawthorn)

Properties: *Western hawthorn* — Heart tonic, vasodilating, hypotensive, antispasmodic, sedative, antidiarrheal. *Chinese hawthorn* — Digestive aid, anthelmintic, circulatory stimulant, antidiarrheal.

Most Common Traditional Uses: *Western hawthorn* — Heart ailments, circulatory disorders (hypertension, arteriosclerosis, etc.), menstrual bleeding, diarrhea. *Chinese hawthorn* — Indigestion, tape worm infections, diarrhea, abdominal pain, colic, enteritis, amenorrhea; also externally for lacquer sores (a form of contact dermatitis), itching and frostbite.

Although the two major types of hawthorn are derived from closely related plants, their uses over the years have diverged into different paths, with only minor overlap.

The traditional uses of Chinese hawthorn are mostly related to the gastrointestinal tract. As children we used to eat candled *shanzha* slices, said to improve the appetite. They were one of our favorite snacks. These are still readily available in Chinese food stores in America. In recent years, it is also used to treat hyperlipemia (high blood lipids). Despite its long use and safety history, it is advisable to exercise moderation (as in everything else) because according to Li Shi-Zhen, the great herbalist (late 16th century), eating too much raw *shanzha* can ruin one's teeth.

Extracts of Western hawthorn in various preparations (oral and injectable) are widely used in Europe as natural drugs for treating heart conditions.

Both types of hawthorn have similar chemical components that include flavonoids, triterpenoids (crataegolic acid, oleanolic acid), vitamins (C, B1, B2), etc. Some of these, especially the flavonoids, have strong pharmacological activities (including beneficial effects on the heart) as well as sedative and antioxidant effects. Since increasing scientific evidence is implicating antioxidants as the next generation of super nutrients, being able to beneficially affect various systems of our body, it is not surprising to see hawthorn, being rich in flavonoids, work in widely different ways.

The use of Chinese hawthorn decoction as a wash to treat lacquer sores (a form of contact dermatitis) and itching dates back to at least the fifth century A.D. This means that the decoction (a hot water extract) must have antiinflammatory, immunomodulating and/or anti-irritant properties. These properties should be useful in cosmetic skin care applications.

References: CHP; JIANGSU; LUST; LEUNG AND FOSTER; ODY; TYLER; WANG 2

HONEYSUCKLE (Syn. *Jinyinhua*)

Plant Source: *Lonicera japonica* Thunb. and other *Lonicera* spp. (Family Caprifoliaceae)

Part Used: Flower buds

Properties: Fever-reducing, detoxifying, antiinflammatory, antiviral, antibacterial

Most Common Traditional Uses: Colds, influenza and associated fevers, swellings, skin sores and boils

Modern/Recent Uses: Bacterial and viral infections, especially pyogenic infections and upper respiratory tract infections, urticaria

Honeysuckle has a special meaning for me. When I was growing up, we used to have our share of colds and flus and associated fevers. My grandmother, being our only family "physician," would go to the local herb shop and bring home a handful of honeysuckle flowers neatly wrapped in paper. She would then boil them to make a strong tea (decoction) which we drank with no complaints. I remember our fever would be gone in no time and we would be out playing again. We never used any modern drugs, not even aspirin.

Numerous species of *Lonicera* are used as sources of honeysuckle. They are found growing either as vines or as erect or climbing shrubs with mildly to highly fragrant flowers. Several of them can now be found wild or in gardens in the United States.

Although one seldom hears about the medicinal uses of honeysuckle in America, its flower and vine are one of the most widely used herbs in China, with a documented use and safety history of two thousand years. It is widely used for treating what traditional Chinese medicine calls "toxic" conditions, such as swellings, sores and boils, as well as food, drug and industrial (pesticide, heavy metal, etc.) poisoning. It is also widely used in China to treat viral and bacterial infections (influenza, sore throat, mumps, bacterial dysentery, enteritis, acute laryngitis, acute mastitis, etc.) and cancers (*e.g.*, angiosarcoma and cancers of the tonsil, bladder and colon). A decoction of the vine has been successfully used to treat infectious hepatitis.

Honeysuckle flower contains up to 12% chlorogenic acid and isochlorogenic acid (coffee contains 5 to 10% chlorogenic acid), flavonoids, saponins and a volatile oil. Leaf and stem contain flavonoids, loganin and secologanin. Chlorogenic acid and the saponins are currently believed to be responsible for most of honeysuckle's effects. In addition, chlorogenic acid has been found to protect experimental animals from substances that cause cancer and to prevent the formation of carcinogens, such as nitrosamines (from nitrites).

The observant reader will have noticed that if chlorogenic acid were indeed responsible for honeysuckle's effects, then coffee should have the same effects due to its high content of this same ingredient. But you are not going to see chlorogenic acid or coffee extract or honeysuckle extract show up as the next "hot" anticancer or antiviral drug for two major reasons. First, as with most modern scientific studies on herbal medicines, these pharmacologic effects are isolated and do not represent those of the herbs, nor are they usually of any practical relevance. And second, even if chlorogenic acid is in fact eventually conclusively proven to be a strong antitumor and antiviral agent, it will be so easy and cheap to produce that under our current drug introduction system, there will be no big profits to provide an incentive to any drug company to manufacture it for your and my benefit.

References: CHP; JIANGSU; LEUNG; LEUNG AND FOSTER; WANG 2

JOB'S TEAR (Syn. Coix seed; Chinese pearl barley; *yiyiren*)

Plant Source: *Coix lachryma-jobi* L. and *C. lachryma-jobi* L. var. *ma-yuen* (Roman.) Staph. (Family Gramineae)

Part Used: Ripe seed

Properties: Diuretic, Spleen-invigorating, heat-dispersing, easing joints, antiswelling, pus-expelling, antioxidant, general tonic

Most Common Traditional Uses: Painful joints, rheumatism, edema

Modern/Recent Uses: Warts, eczema, chronic enteritis, diarrhea, lung abscess, acute appendicitis

Job's tear is commonly used in Asia as a food and a medicine. In China, it is one the most popular food herbs used in the diet therapy of painful and stiff joints, either singly or in soup mixes. From all traditional accounts, it seems to work. If you suffer from stiff and painful joints, I urge you to try this before going the irreversible route of the steroids. Simply cook 1 to 2 ounces as you would regular barley and drink the soup, or eat it all if you prefer. Give it a week or two to take effect. If it doesn't work, you will not have lost anything. If it does, it will have saved you a potential life-long addiction to steroids with the ensuing misery.

Many of the traditional uses of Job's tear may now have a scientific basis. During the past few decades, based on experimental animal studies, Japanese scientists have isolated numerous active chemical components from Job's tear. These include coixol (antiinflammatory, antihistaminic, muscle relaxant, fever reducing, etc.) and coixans (peptide-containing polysaccharides that have sugar-lowering properties). In addition, Job's tear also contains the more common nutrients that have more subtle effects which cannot be meaningfully measured by animal experiments. These nutrients include lipids (glycolipids, phospholipids, sterols, etc.), amino acids, adenosine, thiamine, and others.

Job's tear is also commonly known as Chinese pearl barley in America. After cooking (requiring one hour or more), it does taste like common barley. However, it is different in many respects from regular barley. The latter does not have the reputed effects of Job's tear. Ironically, the common barley has in recent years found its way into soup mixes that are supposed to contain Job's tear. I have come across it numerous times in such mixes sold in American Chinatowns. These adulterated mixes would not yield the benefits of Chinese pearl barley or Job's tear.

References: CHP; JIANGSU; LEUNG AND FOSTER; WANG 2

JUJUBE, COMMON (Syn. Chinese jujube; red date; *hongzao; dazao*)

Plant Source: *Ziziphus jujuba* Mill. and *Z. jujuba* Mill. var. *inermis* (Bge.) Rehd. (Family Rhamnaceae)

Part Used: Dried ripe fruit

Properties: General tonic, normalizes body functions, invigorates *qi* (vital energy), promotes secretion of body fluids, detoxifies, regulates body nutritional balance and defense, tonifies blood, improves complexion

Most Common Traditional Uses: Lack of appetite, fatigue, loose stool, hysteria, dry skin

Modern/Recent Uses: Anemia, hypertension, purpura

The common jujube is one of the most valued Chinese *qi* (*chi*, energy) tonics (also see astragalus). It is often used in Chinese diet therapy with a recorded safe use history dating back to 800 B.C. Reputed to smoothen and moisten the skin to give it a "lustrous" appearance, common jujube is frequently eaten in soups in winter when the skin is dry and itchy.

Common jujube is rich in nutrients, both conventional (vitamins A, B2, C, β-carotene, amino acids, trace minerals, etc.) and non-conventional (flavonoids, sterols, triterpenes, triterpene glycosides, cyclic AMP, etc.), which together are responsible for its beneficial properties.

In an effort to find out why common jujube is so highly valued, scientists have discovered bits and pieces of evidence which may or may not have relevance to its traditional benefits. For example, it has been found to contain the highest concentration of cyclic AMP (adenosine-3',5'-monophosphate) so far discovered in nature. Although cyclic AMP's precise function is not clear, it is involved in numerous critically important life functions, such as serving as a hormonal "messenger." Cyclic AMP has also been speculated to be a major chemical involved in the balancing of the *yin* and *yang*. Scientists have also found that two of common jujube's triterpenes (ursolic acid and oleanolic acid) inhibit the initial step of tooth decay caused by the cariogenic (cavity-producing) bacterium *Streptococcus mutans*. However, these two chemicals are also present in many other fruits and herbs (*e.g.*, ligustrum, mume and olives). Once again, how relevant are these scientific findings? We may never know.

References: CHP; JIANGSU; LEUNG AND FOSTER; WANG 2

JUNIPER

Plant Source: *Juniperus communis* L. (Family Cupressaceae)

Part Used: Dried ripe fruit

Properties: Diuretic, carminative, gastrointestinal antiseptic and irritant, uterine stimulant

Most Common Traditional Uses: Kidney and bladder infections, colic, flatulence, digestive problems

Juniper berry contains a volatile oil which is generally considered to be the active medicinal component. In addition, it contains various nutrients, including flavonoids, sterols, catechins, proanthocyanidins, and fatty acids, many of which have beneficial biological activities, such as antioxidant effects.

Juniper berry is one of the most important flavor ingredients in gin. It is also frequently used to flavor other alcoholic beverages (*e.g.* bitters) as well as nonalcoholic drinks. Despite its contraindications in pregnancy and inflammatory kidney diseases, the amounts of juniper berry present in gin and other alcoholic and nonalcoholic beverages are too low to cause any problems unless one is foolish enough to abuse them. Nevertheless, when used as a medicine in sufficient doses for extended periods of time, one should exercise caution, especially during pregnancy.

References: Leung and Foster; Lust; Tyler

KUDZU (Syn. *Gegen*)

Plant Source: *Pueraria lobata* (Willd.) Ohwi. and *P. thomsonii* Benth. (Family Leguminosae)

Part Used: Root tuber

Properties: Diaphoretic, febrifuge, promotes secretion of body fluids, accelerates eruption of measles, detoxicant, antidiarrheal, thirst quenching

Most Common Traditional Uses: Colds and flus and associated fever and headache, stiff and sore neck, diarrhea, measles, thirst, drunkenness

Modern/Recent Uses: *Internal* — Hypertension, angina pectoris, migraine, diabetes, nasal sinusitis, urticaria, psoriasis, itching. *External* — Traumatic injuries.

The first written record of kudzu in China dates back to the fifth century B.C., and its first recorded medicinal applications date back about two thousand years. The kudzu plant is truly versatile and economic. Its root produces a starch similar to arrowroot starch, which is widely used by Asians (especially Chinese and Japanese) as a food and medicine; the root itself is also eaten in soups or is cooked alone or with other herbs for treating various conditions. Being rich in protein and other nutrients, the whole aboveground portion can be used as animal feed. The fiber from the vine can be used in making textile.

After being introduced into the United States from Asia a little over a hundred years ago, one of the kudzu vines (*Pueraria labata*) has now run wild, especially in the Southeast. There, it overruns telephone poles, abandoned houses and cars, and is considered a pest. Instead of viewing it as a natural resource for use as human and animal food, as medicine and as industrial fiber, our government has been spending money to support program after program trying to eradicate it. What else is new?

I remember when I was growing up, kudzu often showed up on our dinner table in the form of a soup, for what my grandma used to call too much "hot air" among us. In Cantonese folk medicine, "hot or feverish air" or simply "hot" conditions are characterized by one or more of the following: headache with a feeling of heaviness in the head, dryness of mouth, bitter taste in the mouth, bad breath, canker sores, blisters in the mouth, swollen gums, dry and uncomfortable feeling in the throat, bloodshot eyes, pain during urination, etc. Many of these "hot" conditions can now be correlated to viral or bacterial infections. Other foods good for these indications include mung bean, chrysanthemum and watercress. Kudzu root and flower are also used to treat hangovers. Maybe my grandma served kudzu root soup surreptitiously for one of my uncles who was known to hit the bottle once in a while!

References: CHP; Foster and Yue; Jiangsu; Leung and Foster; Wang 1; Wang 2

LICORICE

Plant Source: *Glycyrrhiza uralensis* Fisch. (Chinese licorice) and *Glycyrrhiza glabra* L. (European licorice) [Family Leguminosae]

Part Used: Root and rhizome

Properties: Demulcent, expectorant, antitussive, mild laxative, detoxicant, antioxidant, anti-allergic, antiinflammatory, healing

Most Common Traditional Uses: Gastrointestinal ulcers, sore throat, cough, bronchial problems, food poisoning, abdominal pain, insomnia, sores, abscess

Licorice is perhaps the most widely used herb in the world. Its water extract is extensively used in flavoring foods (especially licorice candy) and tobacco, particularly in Western countries. Licorice is present in many Chinese herbal formulas, most of the time as an adjuvant to bring out the good effects of major herbs or to mitigate some of their undesirable effects. Considering the fact that there are about 100,000 herbal formulas published in Chinese books (64,000 in one work alone), there must be at least another 100,000 not published but used by over 1 billion of the world's population. Just imagine how much licorice is being consumed daily in China alone!

One of the best known uses of licorice is in treating ulcers (*e.g.*, gastric and duodenal). Unfortunately, prolonged use leads to such undesirable effects as potassium depletion, sodium retention, fluid retention and high blood pressure. Up until recently, the active principle was believed to be glycyrrhizin, which is also a sweetening agent; it is also responsible for the above-mentioned side effects. It turns out, however, that glycyrrhizin is not the only active principle in licorice. After removing glycyrrhizin from licorice, researchers found that the deglycyrrhizinated licorice extract is still effective in treating ulcers, but without the toxic side effects of whole licorice. Japanese and Chinese scientists have determined the active principles in the deglycyrrhizinated licorice to be flavonoids. Scientists at the Chinese Academy of Sciences have also found these flavonoids to have very strong antioxidant properties. Thus, in one experiment measuring oxygen free radical scavenging, they found that weight to weight, 1 part of the flavonoids removed almost twice the amount of free radicals that were removed by 100 parts of vitamin E. Based on this single experiment, licorice flavonoids are certainly *the* strongest antioxidants I have ever come across.

Licorice extracts in glycerin or water have very good healing properties which can be used beneficially in skin care cosmetics.

References: CHP; JIANGSU; FOSTER AND YUE; LEUNG; LEUNG AND FOSTER; LUST; WANG 2

LIGUSTRUM (Syn. *Nuzhenzi*)

Plant Source: *Ligustrum lucidum* Ait. (Family Oleaceae)
Part Used: Dried ripe fruit
Properties: *Yin* tonic, brightens vision, darkens hair, invigorates Liver and Kidney, nourishes blood
Most Common Traditional Uses: Premature graying of hair, dizziness, tinnitus, sore back and knees, blurred vision, habitual constipation in the elderly
Modern/Recent Uses: Chronic benzene poisoning

Ligustrum is one of the most highly valued Chinese tonics, often used in soup mixes and wines. In an effort to understand how and why it has been so highly valued since around 800 B.C., Chinese scientists have recently found that it exhibits a wide variety of pharmacological effects both in animals and in humans. These effects include immunomodulating, antiinflammatory, hypolipemic and antiatherosclerotic, hypoglycemic, antimutagenic, anti-allergic, sedative, diuretic, mild cardiotonic, antitumor and the prevention of leukopenia caused by chemotherapy and radiotherapy, etc. Many of these effects are due to oleanolic acid (also present in common jujube) which is present up to 4.3% in ligustrum, the highest among two hundred fifteen herbs tested by Chinese researchers. But oleanolic acid is probably not the only key to ligustrum's function as a highly valued tonic. Some other compounds and nutrients such as ursolic acid, mannitol, fatty acids, glycosides and other still unknown nutrients must also play a role.

According to the great herbalist, Li Shi-Zhen (1590 A.D.), ligustrum also has "beautifying" properties. Maybe for this reason, it is used in hair tonic formulas and formulas for removing facial dark spots primarily intended for internal use. Due to its anti-allergic and antiinflammatory activities, it can be a beneficial ingredient in skin care products.

References: CHP; JIANGSU; LEUNG AND FOSTER; WANG 1; WANG 2

LUFFA (Syn. Luffa sponge)

Plant Source: *Luffa cylindrica* (L.) Roem. and *Luffa acutangula* Roxb. (Family Cucurbitaceae)

Part Used: Fibrous remains of ripe old fruit after removing skin, pulp, seeds, etc.

Properties: Promotes blood circulation, facilitates energy flow in the body, disperses fever, breaks up phlegm, detoxicant, antiinflammatory, analgesic, tranquilizing

Most Common Traditional Uses: Rheumatism, arthritic pain, muscle pain, chest pain, amenorrhea, swollen and painful testicles, hemorrhoids, inadequate milk flow in nursing mothers

Modern/Recent Uses: Shingles

Apart from its usefulness as a bath sponge to remove dead skin tissue and to stimulate the skin, I bet you have never heard of luffa having so many medicinal properties and uses! It certainly doesn't look like it contains more than fibers to do anything to the body besides physical cleansing and stimulation of one's skin. But it has been used in Chinese medicine for at least a thousand years! And some of its uses have recently been substantiated by laboratory findings showing its decoction to have antiinflammatory, analgesic and tranquilizing effects in mice.

Even though we normally associate luffa sponges only with physical actions on the skin, it is perhaps not too far-fetched to envision that some transfer of beneficial ingredients can occur during the physical contact to give the skin extra benefits other than just physical cleansing and stimulation. Thus, its detoxicant and antiinflammatory properties seem to offer some justification for the use of its powder and extracts in facial scrubs and skin cleansers.

References: CHP; JIANGSU; LEUNG; PHILLIPS AND RIX; WANG 2

LYCIUM (Syn. Wolfberry; *gouqizi*)

Plant Source: *Lycium barbarum* L. and *L. chinense* Mill. (Family Solanaceae)

Part Used: Ripe fruit

Properties: *Yin* tonic, improves vision, benefits complexion, nourishes Liver and Kidney, replenishes vital essence (semen), antioxidant

Most Common Traditional Uses: General weakness, lack of energy, aching back and knees, tinnitus, dizziness, diabetes, blurred vision, cough, wet dreams, sexual inadequacies

Modern/Recent Uses: *Internal* — Toxic side effects of chemotherapy and radiotherapy. *External* — Burns, ulcers, bedsores, frostbite, furuncle

One of the best known traditional properties of lycium fruit is its ability to improve vision. This has been documented for over fifteen centuries. Modern scientific studies have finally supplied some substantiation to this property. It turns out lycium fruit not only contains high amounts of β-carotene (8 mg/100 g) but this β-carotene is in a highly biologically active form which is readily utilized by the body.

However, β-carotene is not the only nutrient in lycium fruit, as it is also very rich in amino acids (8 to 10%, half of which are in free form). Also found in lycium are other vitamins (B1, B2, C, nicotinic acid, etc.), polysaccharides that have antioxidant and immunomodulating effects in experimental animals, and other nutrients. Since oral administration of lycium fruit to humans in various studies has also improved their immune functions, raised the serum levels of superoxide dismutase (SOD) and hemoglobin but lowered the level of lipid peroxides and reduced senility symptoms, the polysaccharides obviously are an important active component of lycium fruit. Yet only about 25 years ago, scientists in America were still viewing polysaccharides only as carbohydrates (like starch and sugars) that only supply our body with energy, having no other functions. They were so used to looking for instant responses in their search for fast-acting drugs from nature that they either didn't know how to deal with anything slow-acting or did not have the patience that is normally a characteristic of the Old World. It was only when more and more evidence of these additional properties of polysaccharides kept emerging from Japan, China and Europe that American scientists started to pay attention. Now, they have finally acknowledged that certain carbohydrates (polysaccharides) play important roles in our health other than to simply supply energy.

Another well known and long-documented traditional property of lycium fruit is its ability to "benefit complexion and maintain one's beauty;" it is also considered to have anti-aging properties. To drug-oriented American scientists, this certainly sounds ridiculous. But various studies have shown lycium fruit to have numerous beneficial effects, including antioxidant, immunopotentiating, antimutagenic, hypoglycemic, hypolipemic, hypotensive, etc., all of which contribute to the slowing down of the aging process or helping us live longer. Of course some of the studies are preliminary. But then, what else is not? Many times, you have seen a medical or drug researcher appear on television to announce some "exciting breakthrough," then always end the proclamation with the disclaimer "these results are preliminary and need further studies." Then you never seem to hear from him or her again. The difference between modern drug findings and laboratory studies to verify already well-known and long-standing traditional properties and uses is that the former are based on translating animal responses to humans while the latter are based on already well-known human responses. I would bet on the latter any time.

The "beautifying property" of lycium fruit may have some scientific basis after all, which may justify its use in skin-care cosmetics, as recent laboratory studies not only demonstrated its antioxidant effect but also its ability to increase dermal hydroxyproline level in mice, indicating increased collagen synthesis. All these effects are good for the skin.

References: CHP; Foster and Yue; Jiangsu; Leung and Foster; Zee and Hui; Wang 1; Wang 2

MAGNOLIA (Syn. *Xinyi*)

Plant Source: *Magnolia biondii* L., *M. denudata* Desr. and other *Magnolia* spp. (Family Magnoliaceae)

Part Used: Flower bud

Properties: Clears the nasal cavity, antiinflammatory, anti-allergic, antihistaminic, antimicrobial (fungi, bacteria, viruses), muscle stimulant and relaxant, local anesthetic

Most Common Traditional Uses: *Internal* — Nasal congestion, common cold and associated headache, running nose. *External* — Nasal congestion, toothache, facial dark spots.

Modern/Recent Uses: Allergic rhinitis (*e.g.*, hay fever), chronic rhinitis, paranasal sinusitis

The magnolia flower bud looks like a pussy willow bud, but when crushed it smells strongly of eucalyptus. It is readily available from any Chinatown herb shop. It is one of the most effective nasal decongestants I have ever come across.

I used to have a very bad case of hay fever, both in the spring and fall, all of which started during my third year as a graduate student in Ann Arbor, Michigan. I tried all kinds of over-the-counter and prescription drugs for hay fever. Some worked while others didn't. Those that worked caused drowsiness and made life equally miserable. Later, as my interest in Chinese herbal medicine was rekindled, I discovered magnolia flower and started using it. My hay fever was so bad that my nose was completely plugged at night, and I had to breathe totally through my mouth. When it got *that* bad, none of the modern nasal decongestant drugs worked.

To make the tea, a handful of the buds (8 to 10) are crushed and steeped in boiling water and covered for about 5 minutes. After straining off the hairs, the tea is drunk. Incidentally, it tastes rather bad; only a koala would like it! A cup before bedtime got me through the night. To my amazement, after two seasons of use (once at night and once in the morning whenever I remembered), my hay fever was greatly relieved, to the point that I didn't need any more modern medications. That was a number of years ago. Now I only occasionally need magnolia. Skeptics may say I just happened to be outgrowing my hay fever the same time I started using magnolia flower. Maybe and maybe not. I was also skeptical at first after reading reports from China describing its use in treating rhinitis with amazing results. But the more I read about its history of use and modern studies on its various effects, the more I am convinced that magnolia flower indeed works.

The written record of magnolia flower being used to "clear the nasal cavity" dates back three thousand years. Although modern laboratory studies have discovered various active components (neolignans, lignans, alkaloids, volatile oil, flavonoids, etc.) in magnolia flower, scientists still cannot determine what accounts for its nasal decongestant effects. But as a former regular hay fever sufferer — and still one occasionally — I can only say, "who cares?" I am just glad that I can count on magnolia flower when I need it, even though it makes a horrible tea. To my colleagues and fellow scientists who happen to read this: It is *not just* the volatile oil that works.

Because of its antiinflammatory effects, extracts of magnolia flower are now used in certain cosmetics to relieve irritation or inflammation caused by certain cosmetic ingredients.

References: CHP, Jiangsu; Leung and Foster; Wang 1; Wang 2

MUME (Syn. Smoked plum; *wumei*)

Plant Source: *Prunus Mume* (Sieb.) Sieb. et Zucc. (Family Rosaceae)

Part Used: Oven-dried near-ripe fruit

Properties: Lung and intestinal astringent, promotes secretion of body fluids, expels parasites, anti-allergic, antimicrobial

Most Common Traditional Uses: Chronic cough, chronic diarrhea, diabetes, roundworm and hookworm infections, neurodermatitis, eczema, hard-to-heal sores

Modern/Recent Uses: Allergies (asthma, urticaria, allergic rhinitis, pruritus, etc.), tumors (*e.g.*, polyps)

I first knew mume only as a drink called *suan mei tang* (sour plum drink) which is made by boiling mume in water and then sweetening it with sugar. The drink tastes slightly tart with a hint of smoke flavor (due to processing) and is quite refreshing, especially when drunk in hot weather. It is one of my favorite drinks, and I can now buy it as a syrup concentrate in Chinatown. Later, I discovered mume was also used in a remedy (with licorice and other components) which my grandma sometimes dispensed for sore throat. I never knew that mume had so many other good qualities and uses until I took serious interest in Chinese herbs after I grew up.

Mume is especially effective in treating roundworm and hookworm infections. Also, its extracts have been shown to have antihistaminic and anti-allergic effects in laboratory studies; one of its components, oleanolic acid, may be responsible for part of these anti-allergic effects. Oleanolic acid is also present in the common jujube and other herbs.

Mume extracts are used in skin care cosmetics for their antimicrobial, anti-allergic and healing properties.

References: CHP; JIANGSU; LEUNG AND FOSTER; WANG 2

MUNG BEAN (Syn. Green gram; *ludou*)

Plant Source: *Vigna radiata* (L.) Wilczek var. *ratiata* [*Phaseolus radiatus* L.; *P. mungo* L.; *P. aureus* Roxb.] (Family Leguminosae)

Part Used: Seeds

Properties: Detoxicant, disperses heat, diuretic, hypolipemic

Most Common Traditional Uses: Heat rash, prickly heat, summer heat syndrome (restlessness, irritability, thirst, etc.), heatstroke, food and drug poisoning, "toxic" conditions (erysipelas, carbuncles, boils, swellings, sores, etc.)

Modern/Recent Uses: *Internal* — Agricultural and heavy metal poisoning (*e.g.*, pesticides, lead), mumps, dysentery, enteritis, dyspepsia. *External* — Blackheads, acne, sores, boils, burns.

Although a common food in China, mung bean is often eaten with therapeutic intentions. It is especially popular in summer when it is eaten to prevent heatstroke, heat rash or prickly heat. My favorite way to eat it is mung bean soup sweetened with rock candy and eaten cold.

Mung bean has enjoyed a long history of food and medicinal uses, with a written record dating back to the 10th century A.D. Its best known use is the treatment of poisoning of various types, including foods (*e.g.*, mushroom) and herbal drugs (*e.g.*, aconite). In modern times this use has extended to industrial and environmental poisoning (pesticides, heavy metals, etc.). Some of these treatments have been reported in Chinese herbal and traditional medical journals in recent years.

Mung bean is rich in the traditional nutrients, including protein, carbohydrates, fibers, minerals, vitamins and lipids, among others. It must also be rich in other nutrients so far not yet identified, because the traditional ones just can't explain its detoxifying and heat-dispersing properties.

Based on its effectiveness in treating and healing

burns, reportedly without scars, as well as its recent use in treating acne and blackheads, mung bean flour has found its way into some skin care cosmetics.

One word of caution. Those who cannot tolerate large amounts of fruits and vegetables should avoid eating too much mung bean for long periods.

References: Jiangsu; Leung; Wang 2

PASSION FLOWER

Plant Source: *Passiflora incarnata* L. (Family Passifloraceae)
Part Used: Dried flowering and fruiting tops
Properties: Sedative, antispasmodic, diaphoretic
Most Common Traditional Uses: Insomnia, nervous anxiety, hysteria, nervous headache, neuralgia, epilepsy

Native to the United States, passion flower is one of the best known Western sedative herbs. It is used in many sedative and sleep-aid products in the West, especially in Europe. In fact, the major portion of our production of the herb ends up in Europe, where most of the research and use takes place. Although our own FDA does not recognize passion flower as a safe or effective drug, the German health authorities have approved its use for conditions involving nervous unrest.

Despite continued laboratory studies on passion flower, scientists so far have not yet been able to attribute its medicinal properties to any one single chemical component. Maybe they never will. This applies to most herbs, especially tonics. There is a major flaw in our drug research, production and regulatory control system that prevents adequate and meaningful research to be conducted on herbs. So far, all drug research and approval are based on single chemicals because they are easy to test and control. But research and clinical data in recent years has shown single drugs often are just too toxic or don't work too well. What they should do is start looking at combinations (such as in cancer chemotherapy) and into using tonics to mitigate their toxic side effects as practiced in China. Or better still, treat herbal drugs differently than regular toxic single drugs.

References: Leung and Foster; Lust; Tyler

PEONY, RED AND WHITE [Syn. *Shaoyao; Chishao* (red) and *baishao* (white)]

Plant Source: *Paeonia lactiflora* Pall. (Family Paeoniaceae)

Part Used: *Red Peony Root* — Dried root of wild plant. *White Peony Root* — Cured root of cultivated plant with bark removed.

Properties: *Red Peony Root* — Slightly cold, analgesic, antibacterial, antiviral, antifungal, activates blood, removes blood stasis, detoxicant. *White Peony Root* — Slightly cold, analgesic, antibacterial, antiviral, antifungal, nourishes blood, regulates menstruation, general tonic.

Most Common Traditional Uses: *Red Peony Root* — Tight chest, abdominal pain, "hot" and "toxic" conditions. *White Peony Root* — Tight chest, abdominal pain, headache, dizziness, stiff and painful joints, irregular menses, pale complexion due to blood deficiency, spontaneous perspiration, night sweat.

The peony flower is a symbol of wealth in China and has been part of her classic literature since ancient times.

There doesn't appear to be too much difference between red peony root and white peony root, except that the latter is more commonly associated with use in tonics. The famous Chinese sage Confucius (who lived around 500 B.C.) is said to have favored a sauce made with white peony root. The ancient practice of using peony root as an ingredient in foods and in diet therapy has recently been revived in China. Now, you can find various types of health foods and drinks, including fruit juices, soft drinks (*e.g.*, Shaolin Cola and West Lake Cola), and wines made with extracts of white peony root.

Extracts of both red and white peony roots are also used in skin care cosmetics in China for their antimicrobial, antiinflammatory and astringent properties, especially in acne creams. This use seems to have traditional precedence because its external use to treat carbuncles was recorded in the *Wu Shi Er Bing Fang* (*Prescriptions for Fifty-Two Diseases*) written around 1066 to 771 B.C. This work (a silk scroll copy) was uncovered in 1973 during the excavation of the *Ma Wang Dui* tomb (dated 168 B.C.) at Changsha, Hunan. In the same tomb, numerous herbs were found in sachets clutched in the hand of a skeleton; they included magnolia flower bud, sour jujube kernel, Chinese cinnamon, ginger, and Sichuan peppercorn.

Over the past two decades, Chinese scientists have found red and white peony roots to have various biological activities, including antimicrobial, antiinflammatory, immunomodulating, analgesic, sedative, antispasmodic, antifatigue, antimutagenic, prolonging survival, improving memory, antitumor, etc., in humans and/or experimental animals. They have also discovered that many of these activities are due to the monoterpene glycosides (especially paeoniflorin) present in these herbs. Although these modern findings seem to provide scientific support to some of peony roots' traditional properties and uses, they only represent a fraction of the total properties and uses of these two herbs. In addition, all above effects were results of isolated studies as typical of scientific investigations on herbs. They don't prove anything, but one could interpret these results to one's advantage.

References: CHP; JIANGSU; LEUNG AND FOSTER; LU AND LI; UPHOF; WANG 2

PORIA (Syn. *Fuling*)

Plant Source: *Poria cocos* (Schw.) Wolf. (Family Polyporaceae)

Part Used: Sclerotium (fungal tissue mass)

Properties: Diuretic, nerve-calming, Kidney- and Spleen-invigorating, appetite improving, general tonic

Most Common Traditional Uses: Dysuria (urination difficulties), edema, nervousness, insomnia, forgetfulness, diarrhea, spermatorrhea (wet dreams), cough

With its first written use dating back to around 400 B.C., poria is a widely used tonic food in China, especially for older people. Poria powder is a major ingredient in various *fuling* breads and *fuling* cakes, eaten for their alleged anti-aging effects.

Chemical studies have shown it to contain about 93% of a polysaccharide named β-pachyman along with triterpene acids, sterols, adenine, choline, lecithins and other nutrients. In laboratory studies, scientists in recent years have found the polysaccharide and the triterpene acids to have antitumor and immunoregulatory effects in animals. They also found poria extracts to have sedative and antimutagenic effects. Although isolated and in bits and pieces, these preliminary findings seem to substantiate some of poria's traditional general tonic uses.

Poria is an ingredient in some well-known facial treatment formulas used by women of the Chinese imperial courts. They used it to maintain a clean and "radiant" skin and to prevent pimples, dark spots and wrinkles. Hence it is now used in cosmetics as well.

References: CHP; JIANGSU; LEUNG AND FOSTER; LU AND LI; WANG 2

PURSLANE, COMMON

Plant Source: *Portulaca oleracea* L. (Family Portulacaceae)
Part Used: Aboveground parts
Properties: Heat dissipating, detoxicant, cools blood, stops bleeding
Most Common Traditional Uses: *Internal* — Headache, stomachache, painful urination, dysentery, enteritis, mastitis, lack of milk flow in nursing mothers, postpartum bleeding, bloody stool, bleeding hemorrhoids, metrorrhagia. *External* — Burns, earache, insect stings, inflammations, skin sores, ulcers, pruritus, eczema, abscesses.
Modern/Recent Uses: Colitis, acute appendicitis, diabetes, dermatitis, shingles.

Purslane grows around the world. In addition to being used as a medicine, it is eaten as a vegetable or salad in many countries, especially in France and the Mediterranean. It is rich in nutrients (although amounts are highly variable, depending on the report), including vitamins (A, B1, B2, C, niacinamide, nicotinic acid, α-tocopherol, β-carotene, etc.), fatty acids (especially omega-3 acids, the highest among leafy vegetables), glutathione, flavonoids, coumarins, dopa, dopamine and high concentrations of *l*-noradrenaline (0.25% of fresh herb).

By far the most common medicinal use of purslane in China is for the treatment of dysentery and bleeding. Although modern laboratory studies have shown it to have numerous biological effects such as muscle relaxant (both smooth and skeletal muscles), hypertensive, antibacterial and antifungal, wound-healing, antiinflammatory, uterine stimulant and diuretic, they don't explain why purslane is traditionally used for its various properties.

Nevertheless, since purslane is rich in conventional antioxidants (vitamins A, C and E, β-carotene, glutathione, etc.) and omega-3 fatty acids, and because it has so many traditionally known benefits, it should be utilized more often.

References: CHP; Jiangsu; Leung and Foster; Phillips and Rix; Wang 2

RED SAGE (Syn. *Danshen*)

Plant Source: *Salvia miltiorrhiza* Bge. (Family Labiatae)
Part Used: Root and rhizome
Properties: Activates blood, removes blood stasis, promotes menses, relieves pain, reduces fever, calmative
Most Common Traditional Uses: Blood circulation problems, angina pectoris, palpitations, tight chest, irregular menses, menstrual pain, amenorrhea, metrorrhagia, leukorrhagia, abdominal pain, abdominal mass, insomnia, painful and stiff joints, skin sores, ulcers
Modern/Recent Uses: Chronic hepatitis, coronary heart disease, high blood pressure, stroke, skin diseases (psoriasis, acne, eczema, scleroderma, neurodermatitis, etc.)

The first recorded use of *danshen* dates back at least two thousand years. Considered one of the major *huo xue hua yu* (activating blood circulation to disperse stasis) herbs, it is normally used in teas, wines and sometimes in soups along with rice or other foods/herbs. Modern scientific studies have confirmed many of its traditional properties and uses: cardiovascular, anticoagulant, antibacterial, antiinflammatory, antioxidant, sedative, antiatherosclerotic, antitumor, etc. Its major active ingredients include several tanshinones (phenanthrene diketones), plant acids (salvianolic acid, danshensu, oleanolic acid, etc.), and diterpenoids (miltirone, salvinone); it also contains vitamin E.

Although traditionally used mainly to benefit the cardiovascular system, *danshen* and the isolated tanshinones have recently been successfully used in treating acne, psoriasis, eczema and other skin conditions.

References: CHP; JIANGSU; LEUNG AND FOSTER; WANG 1; WANG 2

REHMANNIA, RAW and CURED (Syn. *Dihuang; sheng dihuang, shu dihuang;* Chinese foxglove)

Plant Source: *Rehmannia glutinosa* (Gaertn.) Libosch. ex Fisch. et Mey. (Family Scrophulariaceae).

Part Used: Dried and/or cured root and rhizome

Properties: *Raw rehmannia* — *Yin* tonic, disperses heat, cools blood, immunomodulating, antitumor. *Cured rehmannia* — *Yin* tonic, warming, tonifies blood, immunomodulating, antitumor, tranquilizing, hypotensive, diuretic, enhances hematopoiesis.

Most Common Traditional Uses: *Raw rehmannia* — Restlessness, thirst, skin eruptions, measles, vomiting blood, nosebleed, diabetes, restless fetus (excessive fetal movement). *Cured rehmannia* — Backache, weak knees, night sweat, spermatorrhea (nocturnal emission), diabetes, palpitations, irregular menses, uterine bleeding, vertigo, tinnitus, premature graying of hair.

Modern/Recent Uses: Rheumatoid arthritis, eczema, urticaria, neurodermatitis (raw rehmannia)

Raw rehmannia is simply the carefully dried root/rhizome, while cured rehmannia is prepared generally by wine curing or by steaming. Wine curing involves mixing the dried rehmannia with wine and steaming in a sealed container until all wine is absorbed; it is then removed, sliced and dried. Steam curing involves steaming the dried rehmannia for hours until the root/rhizome turns black and moist; it is then sliced and dried again.

Both raw and cured rehmannia contain the same type of chemical constituents, including over 25 iridoid, naphthopyrone and phenethyl alcohol glycosides, polysaccharides (especially a fraction named RPS-b), sugars (stachyose, sucrose, etc.), over 15 free amino acids, fatty acid esters, sterols (sitosterol, daucosterol, etc.) and trace minerals. The only difference is the relative proportions of these components, which change as a result of processing. Thus, certain glycosides and amino acids are higher in raw than in cured rehmannia, while simple saccharides (sugars) are higher in cured rehmannia.

Raw and cured rehmannia are often used together in herbal formulations. Both are also commonly used in soup mixes for health maintenance and disease prevention. Although both are *yin* nourishing, raw rehmannia is normally used for febrile conditions while cured rehmannia usually as a blood tonic and for its beneficial effects on the male vital essence (*jing*). The latter is also a common ingredient in hair tonics (for internal consumption) manufactured in China.

Practically all pharmacologic and chemical studies on rehmannia have been done by Chinese and Japanese scientists. They have found considerably more activities than I have listed above, but they have not specified in their reports which rehmannia was tested. For this reason, I have elected not to include them here. Nevertheless, their investigations do seem to provide a scientific rationale for some of the traditional uses of rehmannia, though as usual, the total picture is missing.

Incidentally, don't let the synonym "Chinese foxglove" alarm you. Although rehmannia belongs to the same family as the English foxglove (digitalis — the powerful heart tonic), it does not contain the digitalis cardiac glycosides and its toxicity is as low as many common foods and spices. If you are concerned, you should be more so about drinking diet soda containing the FDA-approved aspartame than consuming an herb/food like rehmannia which has been consumed safely as a tonic food by the Chinese for over two thousand years.[4]

REFERENCES: CHP; JIANGSU; LEUNG AND FOSTER; WANG 1; WANG 2

ROYAL JELLY

Animal Source: *Apis mellifera* L. (honeybee) (Family Apidae)

Part Used: Milky white, viscous substance secreted by worker bees as food for queen bees

Properties: Nutrient, general tonic

Most Common Traditional/Advocated Uses: Malnutrition in children, general weakness in the elderly, chronic hepatitis, diabetes, rheumatism, arthritis, hypertension

The food and medicinal uses of royal jelly appear to be of very recent origin. Hence, unlike ginseng and astragalus, these uses do not have a long historical basis, and only time will tell whether they are indeed valid.

Nevertheless, over the past few decades, there has been considerable chemical and biological work performed on royal jelly. It is very rich in numerous nutrients, including protein, lipids, vitamins, sterols, amino acids, and trace minerals. In addition, it contains 10-hydroxy-*trans*-2-decenoic acid (commonly called 10-HDA), which is generally considered its major active constituent and is thus used in the standardization of royal jelly products. Thus, high-quality frozen royal jelly contains about 2% while freeze-dried powdered royal jelly contains about 5% 10-HDA.

In laboratory studies, 10-HDA has been found to exhibit various biological activities, including antitumor, immunopotentiating, antimutagenic, liver-protectant, antibacterial, antiinflammatory and radiation-protectant effects. Unfortunately, none of these activities can be correlated with a long use history.

One of the most popular uses of royal jelly is in combination with Asian ginseng as an "energizer." Whether royal jelly contributes to the energizing effects of this combination remains to be seen. It is also used in various types of skin-care products for its claimed antiwrinkle and skin-whitening properties.

References: Jiangsu; Leung and Foster

SAFFLOWER (Syn. False saffron; *honghua*)

Plant Source: *Carthamus tinctorius* L. (Family Asteraceae)
Part Used: Flowers
Properties: Invigorates blood, breaks up blood stasis, facilitates menstruation, relieves pain
Most Common Traditional Uses: Cardiovascular problems (amenorrhea, menorrhalgia, coronary heart disease, chest pain, traumatic injuries, etc.)

This herb is the flower of the safflower plant, not the seed, though the latter is also used, for example, in producing safflower oil.

Safflower has been used in China for at least twenty-three centuries. It is one of the major *huo xue hua yu* (activating circulation to dissipate blood stasis) herbs. It contains a complex mixture of red and yellow pigments chemically called chalcones, along with flavonoids, flavonoid glycosides, polysaccharides, lignans, fatty acids and others.

Scientists have found safflower extracts to have various effects on the immune system (both immunosuppressive and immunopotentiating) and the cardiovascular system (anticoagulant, cardiac stimulant, vasodilating, hypolipemic, hypotensive, etc.), with very low toxicity. So far, a yellow pigment (called "safflower yellow") and a polysaccharide have been found to be pharmacologically active in the laboratory. All these only indicate that the traditional uses of safflower do in fact have some scientific basis.

Safflower extracts are now used in hair tonics (*e.g.*, some Chinese hair growth liniments) and facial and body massage and bath preparations, often together with red sage, for their blood-invigorating and vasodilating effects. The idea is that safflower will help open up the capillaries of the skin to facilitate the absorption and utilization of other active herbs in the formula. Safflower is also used as a natural coloring agent, yielding a light yellow to orange color.

Although safflower is also used to "calm" live fetuses and abort dead ones, it is traditionally cautioned against use in pregnancy. However, that only applies to therapeutic doses (*i.e.*, 3 to 6 g and over). In comparison, normal intake from cosmetics (through skin absorption) is minute.

References: JIANGSU; LEUNG AND FOSTER; WANG 2

SARSAPARILLA

Plant Source: Various *Smilax* species. (Family Liliaceae)
Part Used: Dried root and rhizome
Properties: Tonic, carminative, diaphoretic, diuretic, detoxicant, purifies blood, antiinflammatory, liver-protectant
Most Common Traditional Uses: Rheumatism, gout, colds, fevers, inflammations, flatulence, gonorrhea, syphilis, skin disorders (sores and boils), mercury poisoning

There are several types of sarsaparilla derived from different *Smilax* species, depending on the region from which they come: Mexican sarsaparilla (*S. medica* Schlecht.), Honduran sarsaparilla (*S. regelii* Killip et Morton and *S. officinalis* Kunth), Ecuadorian sarsaparilla (*S. febrifuga* Kunth and other *Smilax* spp.) and Jamaican sarsaparilla (*S. regelii*). In addition, some Chinese *Smilax* species are also used, including *S. sieboldi* Miq. and *S. glabra* Roxb.

Sarsaparilla has recently gained a lot of attention as an ingredient in performance-enhancing and anabolic supplements aimed at athletes and body-builders. It appears that some marketer must have hit on the idea that since sarsaparilla is rich in steroids, it should serve as a source of anabolic steroids which are no longer allowed to be used. Unfortunately, there is not the slightest evidence that the human body can turn these sarsaparilla-derived steroids into anabolic steroids. On the other hand, if it were used with the intention of helping the body deal with aches and pains due to excessive physical exercise, there might be some justification due to its traditional use for rheumatic and arthritic pain in different countries. In any case, except for the fact that its saponins (steroid glycosides) may increase the absorption of other drugs taken simultaneously, sarsaparilla is generally nontoxic. Its presence in the above products may not do anything for the consumer; it won't do harm either.

References: JIANGSU; LEUNG AND FOSTER; LUST; TYLER

SAW PALMETTO (Syn. Sabal)

Plant Source: *Serenoa repens* (Bart.) Small. (Family Palmaceae)

Part Used: Ripe fruit

Properties: Diuretic, expectorant, sedative, uterine and vaginal tonic, antiinflammatory, estrogenic and antiestrogenic, antiandrogenic

Most Common Traditional Uses: Inflamed and enlarged prostate, colds, head colds, migraine, coughs, irritated mucous membrane, chronic cystitis, sore throat, asthma, chronic bronchitis, cancer

Other Advocated Uses: Underdeveloped breasts in females, lack of sex vigor and low sperm production in males

Although primarily grown in the United States, most of the saw palmetto berries produced here go to Europe (especially Germany) where the berries are extracted to yield a fat-soluble remedy to treat benign prostatic hyperplasia (BPH) or enlargement of the prostate gland. This is approved by the German government but not by our FDA. If you want this product you may have to go to Germany for it.

Again, as with other herbs, drug-oriented researchers have been trying to pinpoint the single active principle of saw palmetto without much success. Instead, as usual, they have found bits and pieces of evidence. For example, the berries contain β-sitosterol which has some estrogenic activity, but not much. Then again, it also has antiestrogenic effects, which seems to even the score. Furthermore, β-sitosterol is also present in many herbs and foods; hence it is hardly unique to saw palmetto. The fat-soluble fraction has antiandrogenic activity. Some antiinflammatory activity has also been observed, but not enough to account for its effect in BPH. Remember, all these studies were undertaken just trying to find out what makes saw palmetto work on BPH. Try to figure out how saw palmetto works in the alleged breast enlargement and male sex vigor areas? Forget it!

References: LEUNG AND FOSTER; LUST; TYLER

SCHISANDRA (Syn. *Wuweizi*)

Plant Source: *Schisandra chinensis* (Turcz.) Baill. and other *Schisandra* spp. (Family Schisandraceae)

Part Used: Dried ripe fruit

Properties: Lung astringent, Kidney tonic, male tonic, adaptogenic, detoxicant, antimutagenic, antioxidant, liver protectant, central stimulant, tranquilizing

Most Common Traditional Uses: Cough, asthma, involuntary seminal discharge, impotence, insomnia, neurasthenia, chronic diarrhea, night sweat, spontaneous sweating, physical exhaustion, excessive urination

Modern/Recent Uses: Liver diseases

Schisandra is known as *wuweizi* (five-flavored seed) in Chinese because it tastes simultaneously sweet, sour, bitter, salty and pungent when chewed. In addition to its use as a medicine, it is also used as an ingredient in soup mixes.

Schisandra is one of those Chinese herbs without much adequate published English information even though there are many published reports on it in Chinese and Japanese.

It is a well-known tonic, especially for the male. Modern laboratory studies have found some of its constituents (*e.g.*, lignans) to have strong antioxidant and liver-protectant properties. Its extracts and lignans are now being used to effectively treat liver diseases (*e.g.*, viral hepatitis). In the West, silymarin (from milk thistle) is well known for its beneficial effects on the liver. One can soon add schisandra as its equal or superior.

A typical tonic like ginseng, schisandra's actions in the body are subtle. They cannot be readily duplicated in the laboratory. The antioxidant and liver protectant effects of schisandra just mentioned only give you an isolated glimpse of its various pharmacological effects. Believe me, there are too many to list here!

References: CHP; JIANGSU; LEUNG AND FOSTER; TYLER; WANG 1; WANG 2

SESAME

Plant Source: *Sesamum indicum* DC. (Family Pedaliaceae)
Part Used: Black seeds
Properties: Tonic, vitalizes the internal organs, particularly beneficial to the Liver and Kidney, moisturizes and lubricates the intestines
Most Common Traditional Uses: *Internal* — Constipation, dizziness, blurred vision, tinnitus (imaginary roaring noise) resulting from anemia, premature graying of hair, loss of hair after an illness, lack of milk in nursing mothers, rheumatoid arthritis, paralysis, general weakness after an illness. *External* — Insect bites, sores, carbuncles, hemorrhoids, burns, toothache, swollen gums.

In traditional Chinese medicine, black sesame seed is considered superior to the white variety. It has been used by the Chinese for at least two thousand years. Although also a common food, it is regarded by the Chinese as a tonic, beneficial to the hair and internal organs. It is commonly eaten as a soup (thin paste) either sweetened or salted to regulate bowel movement, and for other functions.

The expressed oil of the unroasted seed does not have much of an odor and is used in cosmetic and pharmaceutical formulations for its lubricant effects. The oil from the roasted seed, however, is very fragrant and is the sesame oil so familiar in Chinese foods.

References: CHP; Jiangsu; Leung; Wang 2

SOUR JUJUBE KERNEL (Syn. Sour date kernel; *suan zao ren*)

Plant Source: *Ziziphus spinosa* Hu and *Z. jujuba* Mill. var. *spinosa* (Bge.) Hu ex H.F. Chow (Family Rhamnaceae)
Part Used: Seed
Properties: Brain tonic, tranquilizing, promotes secretion of body fluids, stops excessive perspiration
Most Common Traditional Uses: Neurasthenia, insomnia, nightmares, night sweat, forgetfulness, palpitations, thirst

Sour jujube kernel is probably the most commonly used sedative herb in China for treating sleep-related problems such as insomnia and nightmares. Its first recorded use dates back two thousand years. Since then, it has become a major ingredient of Chinese sedative and hypnotic formulas, some of which are well known and can be obtained over the counter in Chinese herb shops throughout the world.

Sour jujube kernel is also used in soups and drinks for diet therapy. One recipe for rice soup in *Yin Zhan Zhen Yao* (a diet herbal published in 1330 A.D.) simply calls for cooking 100 g of rice to form a soup and then adding 15 g of roasted sour jujube kernel powder shortly before serving. It is said to be good for palpitations, insomnia, excessive dreams (nightmares) and tightness of the chest.

Sour jujube kernel contains a wide variety of chemical components, including flavonoids, flavonoid glycosides, triterpenes and triterpene saponin glycosides, alkaloids, sterols, fatty acids, cyclic AMP and cyclic GMP and others. Modern scientific studies have shown it to have strong sedative and hypnotic effects in both humans and in experimental animals (mice, rats, guinea pigs, cats, rabbits and dogs). As with most drug-oriented modern scientific studies on herbs, no one single active principle has been found. Rather, the flavonoid glycosides (spinosin, swertisin and zivulgarin), alkaloids and the saponins (jujubosides A and B) have all been shown to be active. Perhaps that is the reason sour jujube kernel has been safely and effectively used for over two thousand years!

References: CHP; Jiangsu; Leung and Foster; Lu and Li; Wang 2

THYME (Syn. Garden or common thyme)

Plant Source: *Thymus vulgaris* L. (Family Labiatae)
Part Used: Leaves and flowering tops
Properties: Anthelmintic, antispasmodic, bronchiospasmolytic, carminative, sedative, diaphoretic, expectorant.
Most Common Traditional Uses: *Internal* — Throat and bronchial problems (acute bronchitis, laryngitis, whooping cough), diarrhea, chronic gastritis, lack of appetite. *External* — Neurasthenia, rheumatic problems, paralysis, bruises, swellings, sprains, shingles.

Thyme contains 0.8 to 2.6% of a volatile oil called "thyme oil" which is generally considered its major active component. The oil is composed of various phenols, monoterpene hydrocarbons, alcohols and other volatiles, including thymol and carvacrol. Apart from thyme oil, thyme also contains tannin, flavonoids, triterpenes (ursolic acid and oleanolic acid), phenolic acids (caffeic and labiatic) and other biologically active nutrients. Ursolic acid and oleanolic acid are known to have various biological activities (see common jujube, ligustrum and mume).

Thymol has antispasmodic, expectorant, carminative, anthelmintic (esp. hookworm) and antimicrobial (bacteria and fungi) effects and is used in mouthwashes and toothpaste for its antiseptic properties. But it is also very toxic if accidentally ingested, although not in the amounts usually used in the above products. Just don't drink your mouthwash!

To give thyme a little more credit as a good herb, laboratories have shown thyme oil, thymol and labiatic acid all to have antioxidant properties.

References: LEUNG; LEUNG AND FOSTER; LUST

TURMERIC

Plant Source: *Curcuma longa* L. (Syn. *C. domestica* Val.) (Family Zingiberaceae)
Part Used: Cured and polished rhizome
Properties: Breaks up blood stasis, promotes and normalizes energy flow, relieves pain, antioxidant, antiinflammatory
Most Common Traditional Uses: *Internal* — Flatulence, liver problems, menstrual difficulties, bloody urine, hemorrhage, toothache, traumatic injuries, bruises and sores, chest pain, rib pain, colic, swelling, abdominal mass. *External* — Pain and itching resulting from sores and ringworm infections.

Turmeric is a familiar spice in many Asian dishes, especially Indian (*e.g.*, curry). It is used as much for its flavor as for its intense yellow color. During the past few decades, laboratory studies have shown it to promote bile secretion, increase appetite, lower blood pressure, alleviate pain, stimulate the uterus, reduce inflammation and edema and to have antiinflammatory, antioxidant, antibiotic, insecticidal, antispasmodic, hypocholesterolemic, antimutagenic, antitumor and other activities.

The yellow coloring substance present in turmeric, called "curcumin," appears to be the major active component. But it does not account for all of turmeric's properties. And there you have it again! Lots of bits and pieces of scientific findings but not much proof of anything.

I don't want to criticize my research colleagues, but let's face it! Research money is always difficult to come by. One makes the best out of what one has. Thus, the simplest and cheapest way to accomplish a research project in herbal drugs is to isolate a chemical from any herb and do some preliminary biological testing on it, or simply test an extract of the herb for a specific biological activity. Then, one can publish a research paper reporting that such-and-such active component or fraction has been found in this or that herb and using whatever new biochemical or pharmacological theory or hypothesis is in vogue at that moment, speculate on how this "active principle" correlates to the herb. Of course, 99.99% (my exaggeration) of the time this finding has nothing to do with what that particular herb's properties and functions are. That's why you have all these so-called modern scientific studies that haven't proven the effectiveness of any herb one way or the other. All we have are piles and piles of isolated data that may "indicate" only "some" activity of some herbs. Incidentally you can find some effective single-chemical *drugs* based on all these data. The reason it hasn't been done in the West is because of our drug research and development and government approval system which offers no incentive to produce inexpensive new drugs.

References: CHP; JIANGSU; LEUNG; LEUNG AND FOSTER

WATERCRESS

Plant Source: *Nasturtium officinale* R. Br. (Family Cruciferae)

Part Used: Whole herb

Properties: Diuretic, expectorant, stimulant, stomachic, soothes the lungs, dissipates heat, detoxicant

Most Common Traditional Uses: *Internal* — Tuberculosis, gout, digestive disturbances, anemia, eczema, canker sore, swollen gums, bloodshot eyes, pain during urination. *External* — Skin blemishes, freckles.

Watercress is native to Europe and has been naturalized in America. Westerners usually use it fresh while the Chinese almost always use it cooked. It is considered by Western herbalists as a good source of vitamins, especially C. But once cooked, most of the vitamins are destroyed. Whatever benefits the Chinese believe the herb has must come from some other ingredients.

Watercress was only introduced into China a little over a hundred years ago from America. There is a poignant story behind its introduction. When railroads were being built in California, much of the labor was supplied by Chinese coolies, most of whom came from villages in Guangdong in southern China, where my mother's family lived for generations. San Francisco used to be called *gum san*, which means "golden mountain" in Cantonese. Many Chinese young men were attracted by the idea of fame and fortune in faraway "golden mountain" and headed to America with great hopes. Once they landed in San Francisco, they were carted off to work on the railroad. Under the adverse working conditions, many of them died from tuberculosis or other causes, and never made it home with their fortunes. Some of those who returned home brought with them a new herbal drug. Legend has it that some of the laborers found out that the watercress growing along the streams in the California Sierra was good for their illness, tuberculosis. They started gathering and eating it.

After their ordeal, and with every hard-earned cent saved, they headed home, bringing with them seeds of what they considered a miraculous plant, watercress. Maybe that is the reason this vegetable is so popular among the Cantonese.

The Cantonese consider watercress to have heat-dissipating and detoxifying properties and use it to treat what they call "hot" conditions such as canker sores, swollen gums, bloodshot eyes, pain during urination, dryness of throat and dry cough.

References: JIANGSU; LEUNG; LUST; ZEE AND HUI

REFERENCES

Cheung, S.C. and N.H. Li, Eds. 1978, 1981, 1983, 1985, 1986. *Chinese Medicinal Herbs of Hong Kong.* 5 vols. Commercial Press. Hong Kong.

Chinese Pharmacopeia Committee (CHP), Chinese Ministry of Health. 1990. *Chinese Pharmacopeia*. People's Health Publications. Beijing, PRC. (In Chinese)

Foster, S. and J.A. Duke. 1990. *A Field Guide to Medicinal Plants: Eastern and Central North America.* Houghton Mifflin Co., Boston, MA.

Foster, S. and C.X. Yue. 1992. *Herbal Emissaries.* Healing Arts Press. Rochester, VT.

Jiangsu Institute of Modern Medicine. 1977. *Encyclopedia of Chinese Materia Medica.* 2 vols. Shanghai Scientific and Technical Publications. Shanghai, PRC. (In Chinese)

Leung, A.Y. 1984. *Chinese Herbal Remedies.* Universe Books. New York, NY. [Republished as: *Chinese Healing Foods and Herbs.* AYSL Corp. 1993. Glen Rock, NJ]

Leung, A.Y. and S. Foster. 1995. *Encyclopedia of Common Natural Ingredients Used in Food, Drugs and Cosmetics.* 2nd Ed. John Wiley and Sons. New York, NY. (In Press)

Lu, Q.Y. and M. Li. 1987. *Chinese Herbs for Life Extension.* People's Health Publications. Beijing, PRC. (In Chinese)

Lust, J.B. 1974. *The Herb Book.* Benedict Lust. Simi Valley, CA.

Ody, P. 1993. *The Complete Medicinal Herbal.* Dorling Kindersley. New York, NY.

Peng, Q.M. 1987. *Comprehensive Treatise on Chinese Medicinal Foods.* Sichuan Scientific and Technical Publications. Chengdu, PRC. (In Chinese)

Phillips, R. and M. Rix. 1993. *Vegetables.* Random House. New York, NY.

Richardson, J. 1981. *Wild Edible Plants of New En-*

gland. The Globe Pequot Press. Chester, CT.

Tyler, V.E. 1987. *The New Honest Herbal*. George F. Stickley Co. Philadelphia, PA.

Uphof, J.C.T. 1968. *Dictionary of Economic Plants*. J. Cramer Stechert-Hafner. New York, NY.

Wang, Y.S. *et. al.* (WANG 1), Eds. 1983. *Pharmacology and Applications of Chinese Materia Medica*. People's Health Publications. Beijing, PRC. [English translation: Chang, H.M. and P.P. But. 1986. *Pharmacology and Applications of Chinese Materia Medica*. World Scientific. Hong Kong.]

Wang, Z.Y. *et. al.* (WANG 2), Eds. 1992. *Encyclopedia of Chinese Herbal Foods*. Dalian Press. Dalian, PRC. (In Chinese)

Zee, S.Y. and L.H. Hui. 1981. *Hong Kong Food Plants*. The Urban Council. Hong Kong.

1. Anon. 1994. Congress Investigates FDA Links to Monsanto. *Natural Food Merchandiser. June:* 3 and 14.

2. Salaman, M.K. and J.V. Wright. 1994. Would You Buy a Used Car from FDA? *Townsend Letter for Doctors. August/September:* 968-973

3. Siegel, R.K. 1979. Ginseng Abuse Syndrome, Problems with the Panacea. *JAMA. 241:* 1614-1615.

4. McCaleb, R.S. 1993. Food Ingredient Safety Evaluation. *HerbalGram. 29*: 40-44.

5. Cui, N.X. 1990. Fresh Ginger Juice in the Treatment of 19 Cases of Burn Patients. *Zhejiang Journal of Traditional Chinese Medicine. (10):* 451.

Herbs and Foods

Color Plates

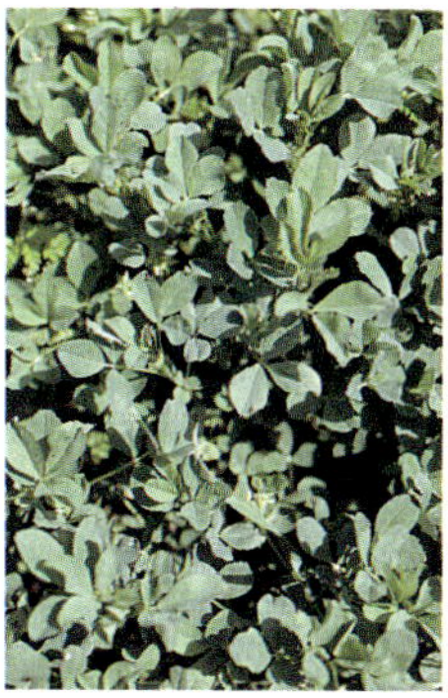

Alfalfa
(Medicago sativa)

苜蓿

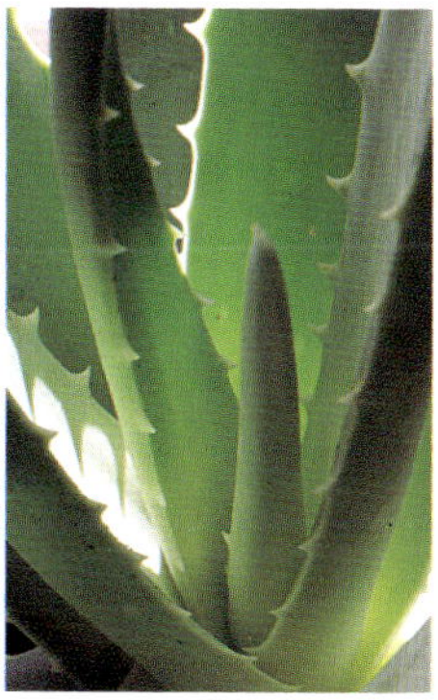

Aloe Vera
(Aloe barbadensis)

芦荟

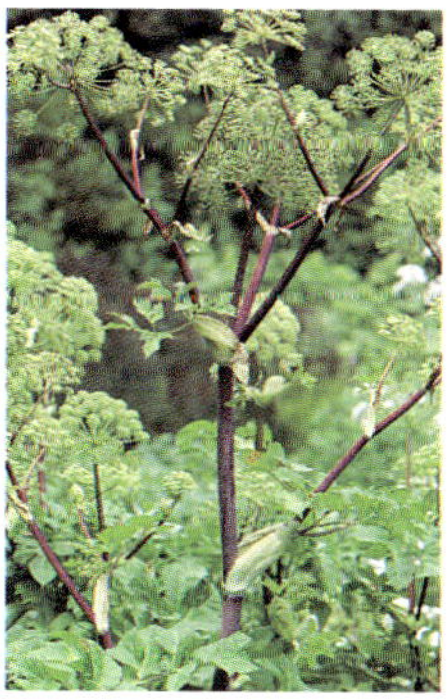

Angelica
(Angelica archangelica)

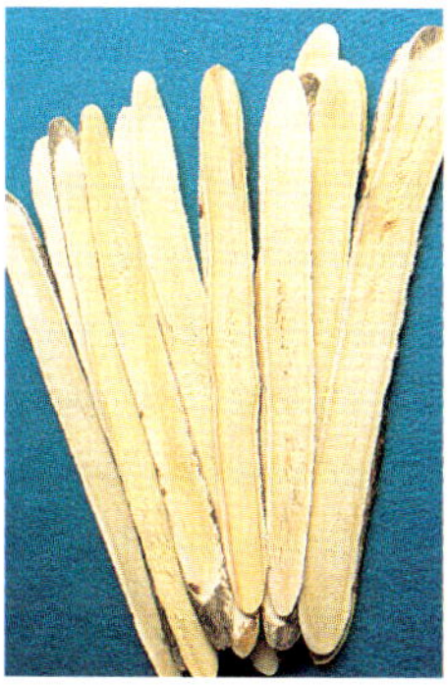

Astragalus

黄芪

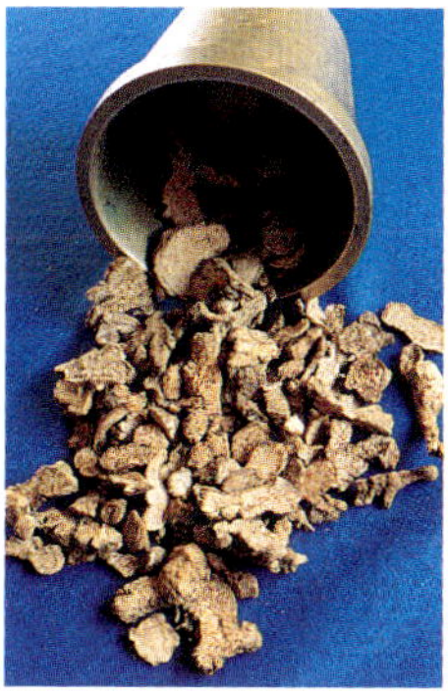

Baizhu

白术

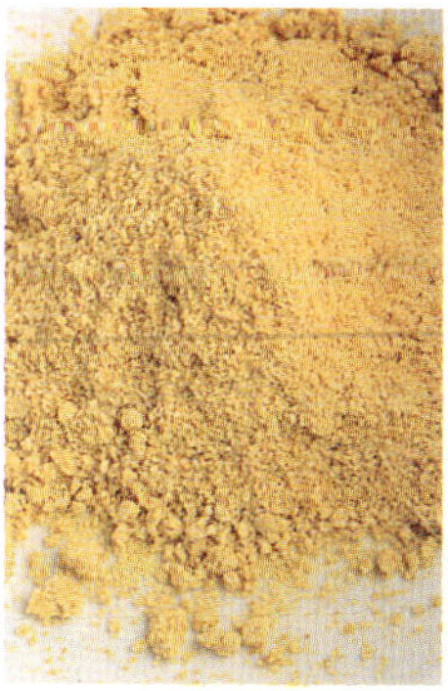

Bee Pollen

花粉

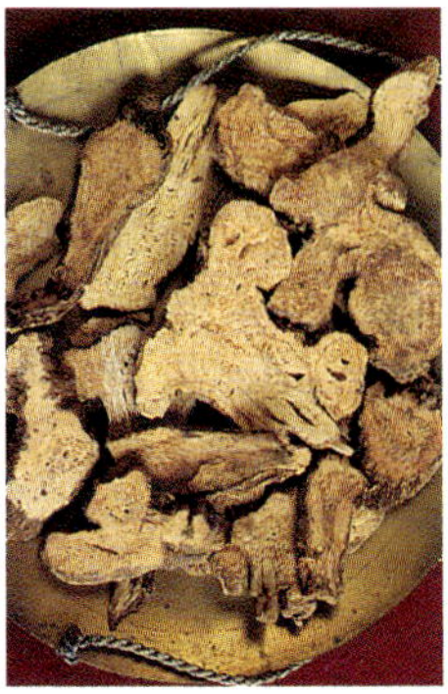

Cangzhu

苍术

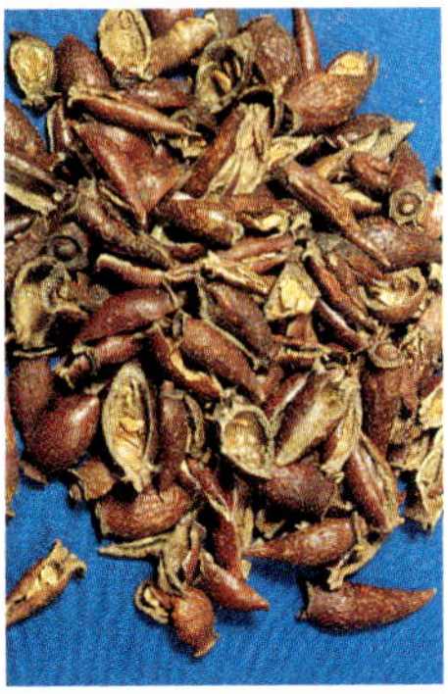

Cherokee Rosehip

金樱子

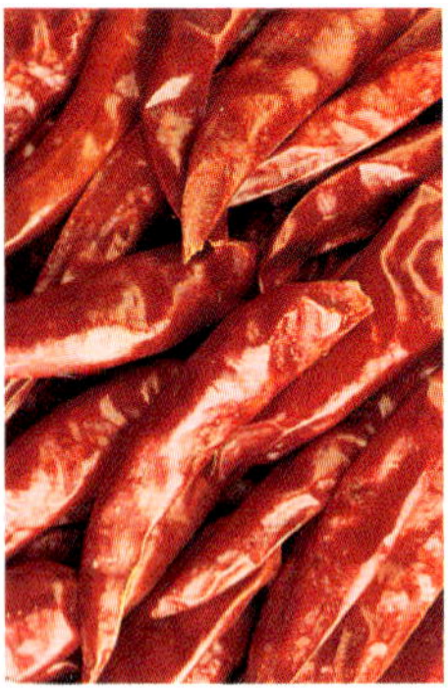

Capsicum

辣椒

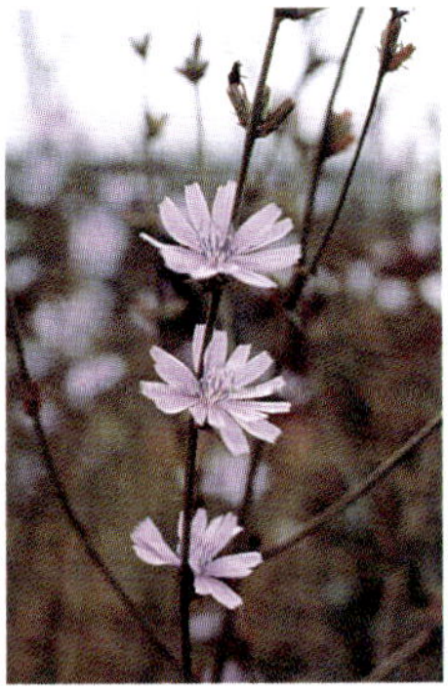

Chicory *(Cichorium intybus)*

菊苣

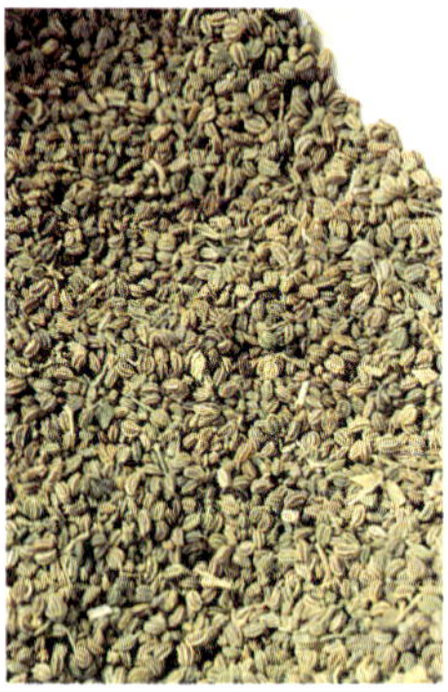

Celery Seed

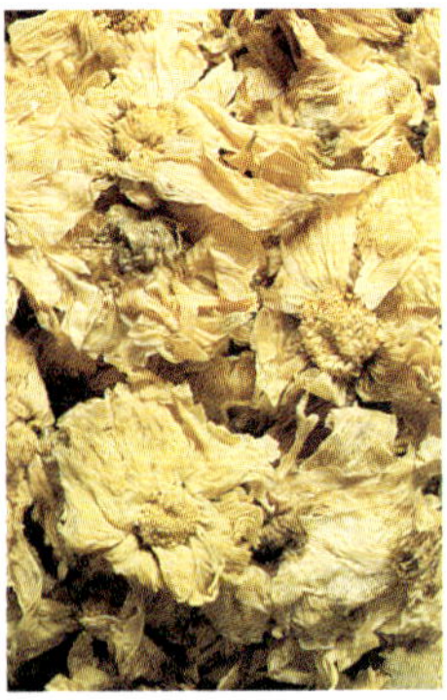

Chrysanthemum

菊花

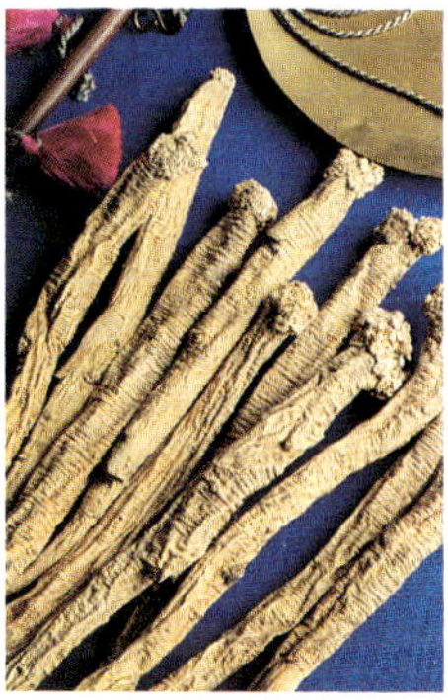

Codonopsis

党参

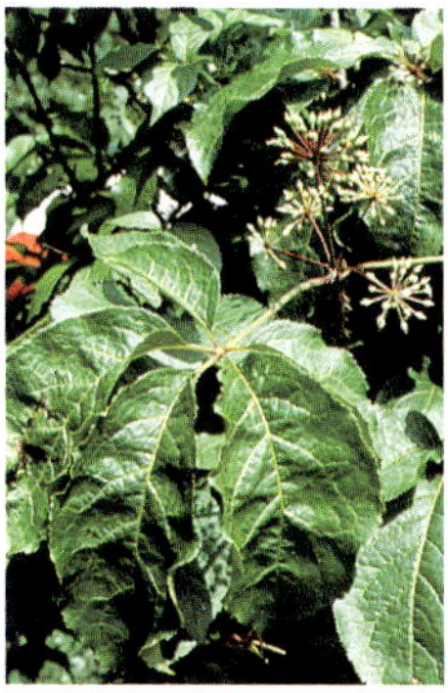

Eleuthero
(Eleutherococcus senticocus)

刺五加

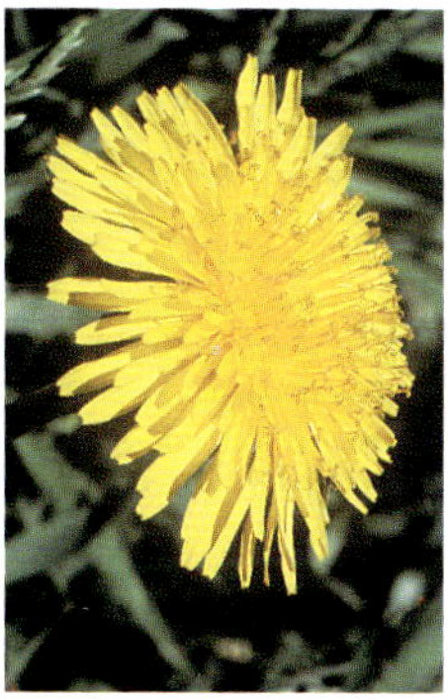

Dandelion
(Taraxacum officinale)

蒲公英

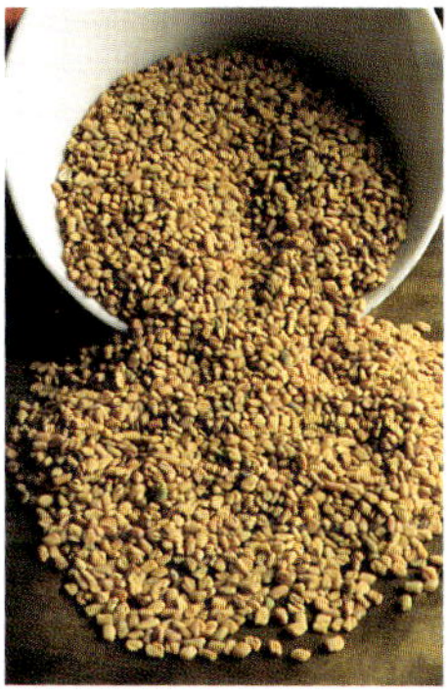

Fenugreek

胡芦巴

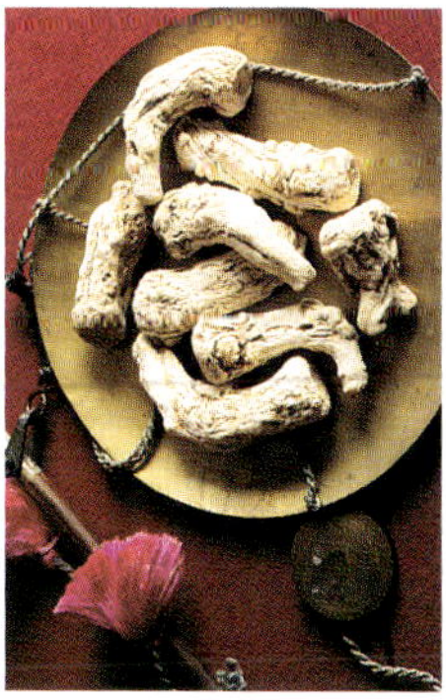

Danggui

当归

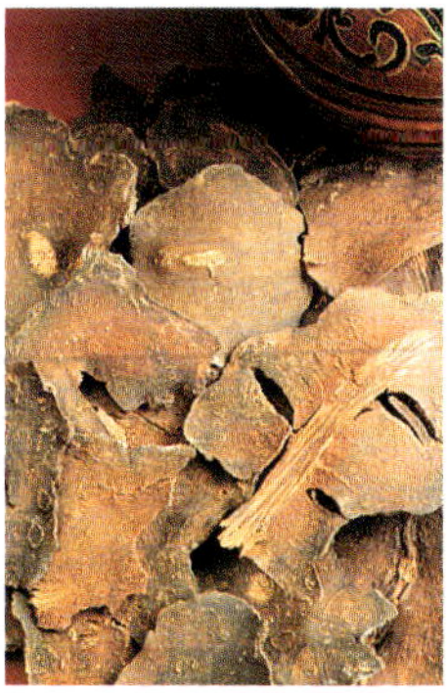

Fo-ti, Cured

何首乌

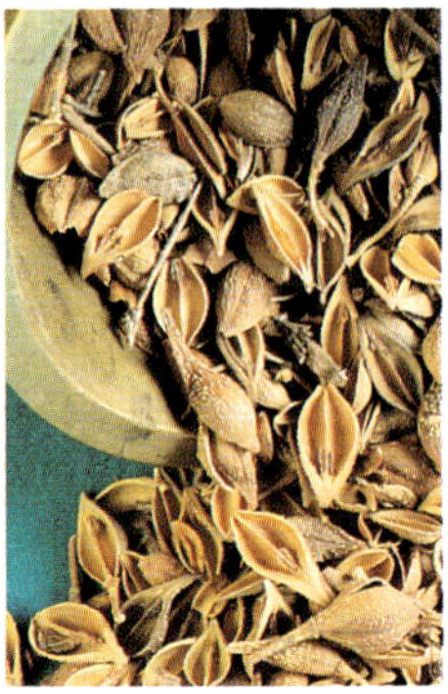

Forsythia

连翘

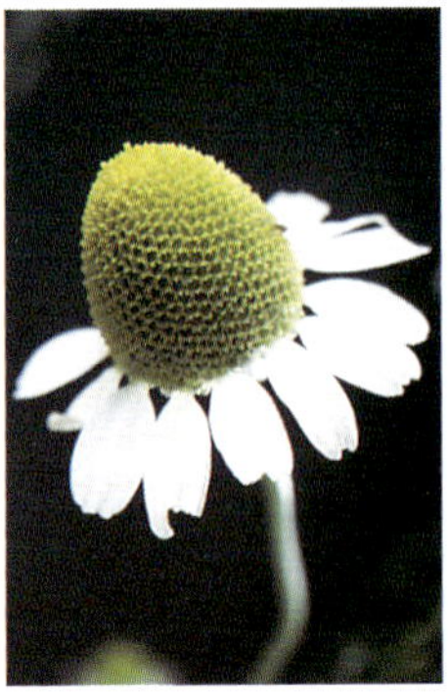

German Chamomile *(Matricaria recutita)*

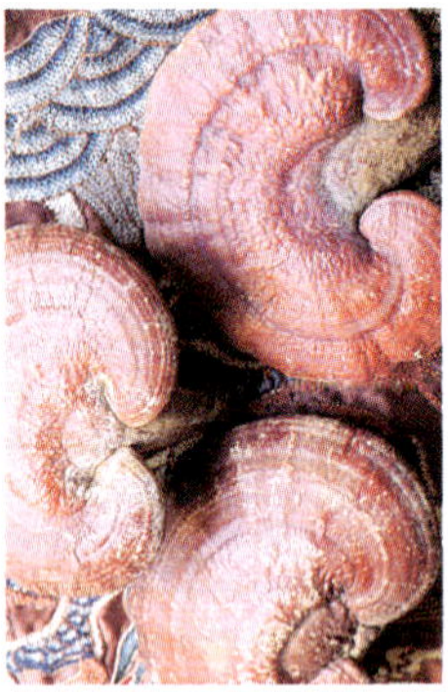

Ganoderma

灵芝

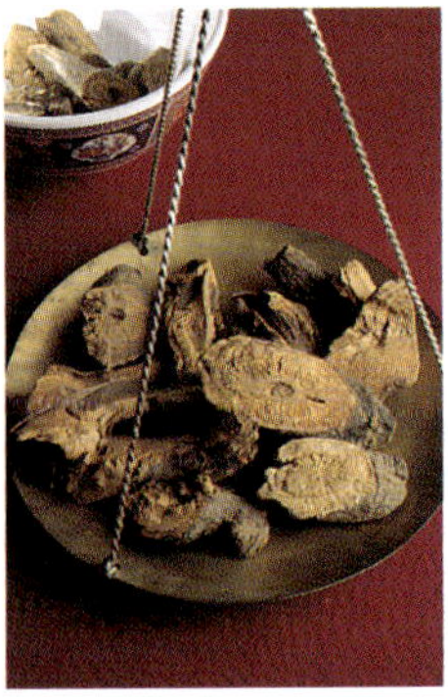

Giant Knotweed

虎杖

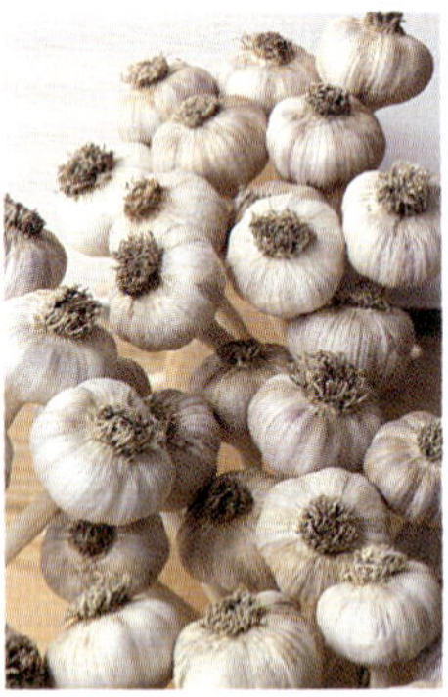

Garlic

大蒜

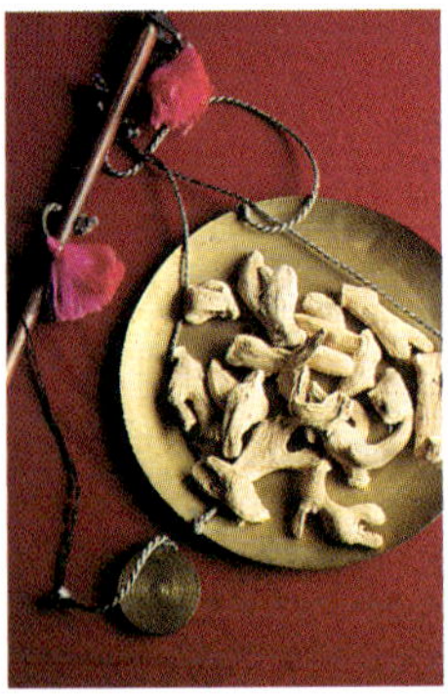

Ginger

姜

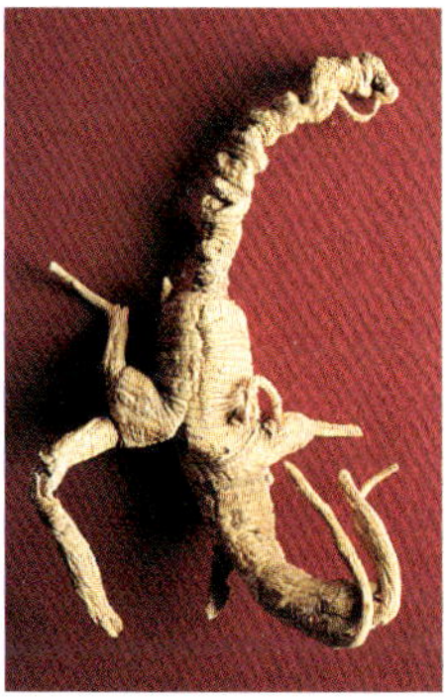

Ginseng, American

西洋参

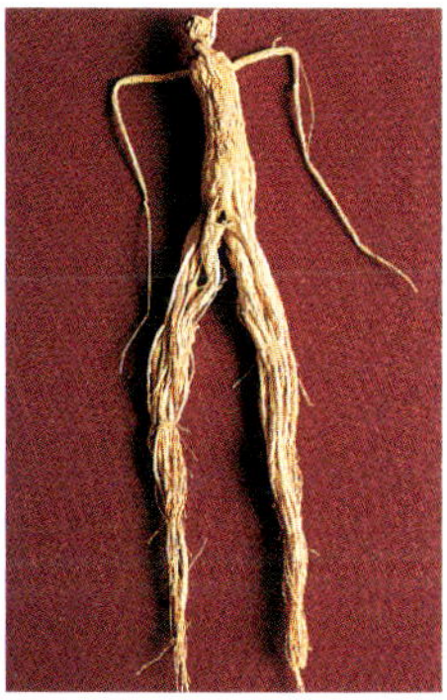

Ginseng, Asian

人参

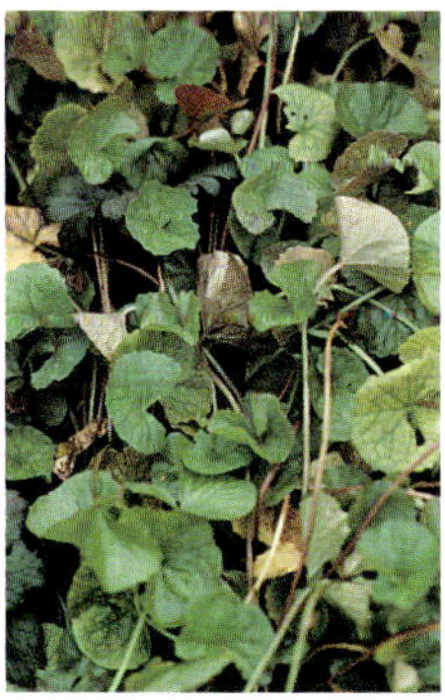

Gotu-kola
(Centella asiatica)

積雪草

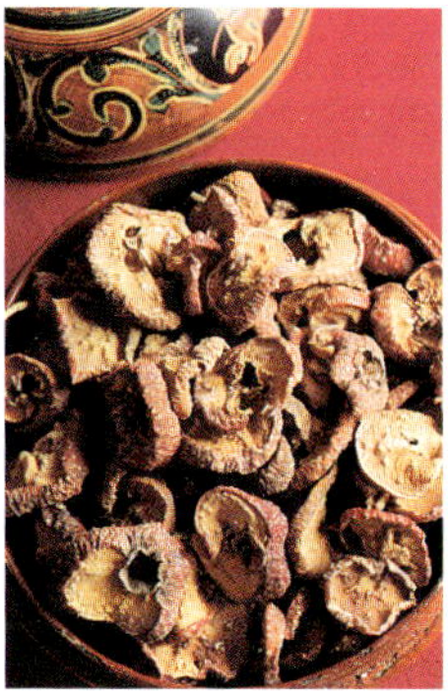

Hawthorn, Chinese

山楂

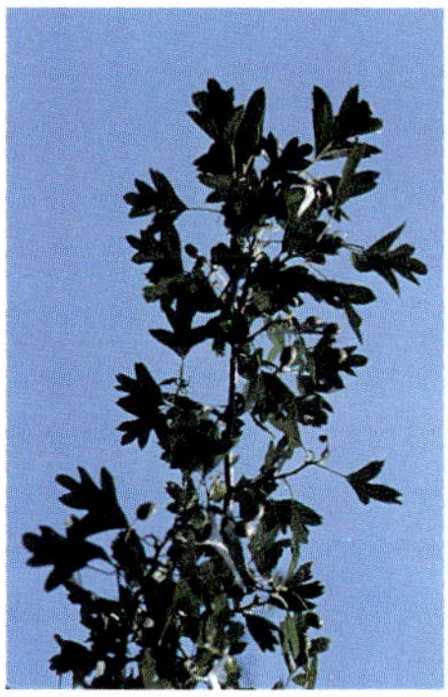

Hawthorn, Western
(Crataegus laevigata)

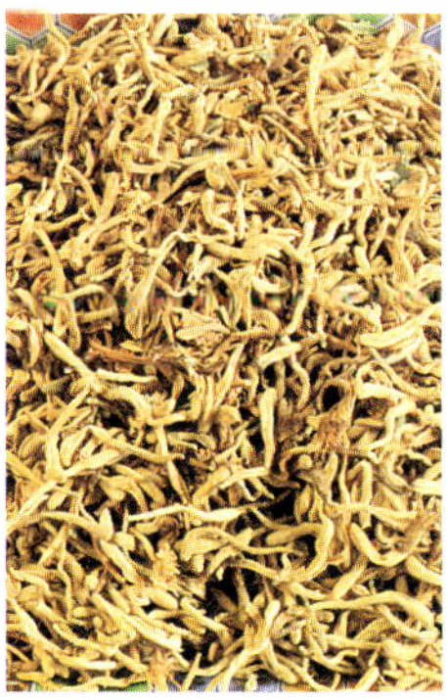

Honeysuckle

金银花

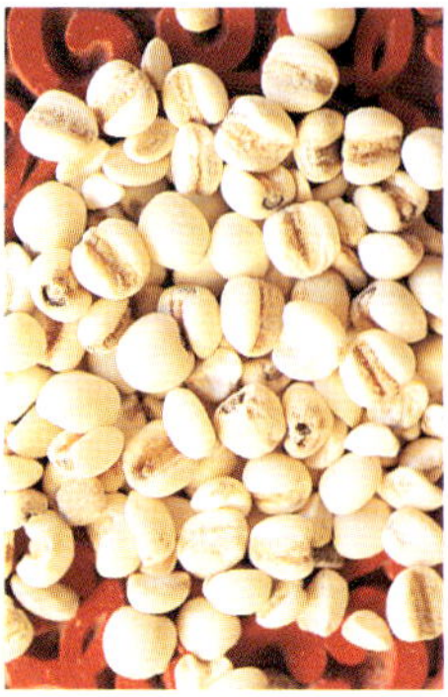

Job's Tears

薏苡仁

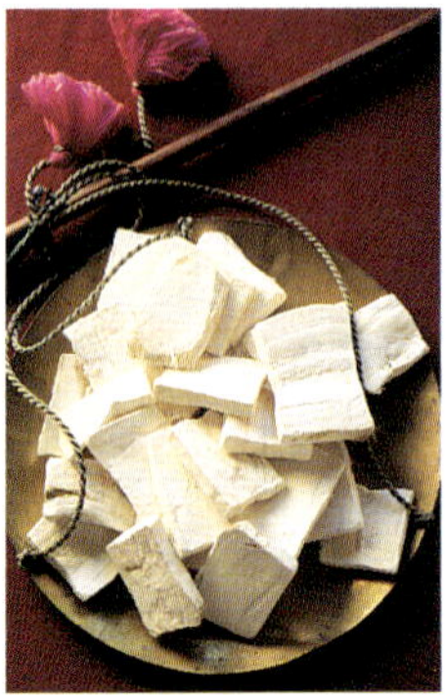

Kudzu

葛根

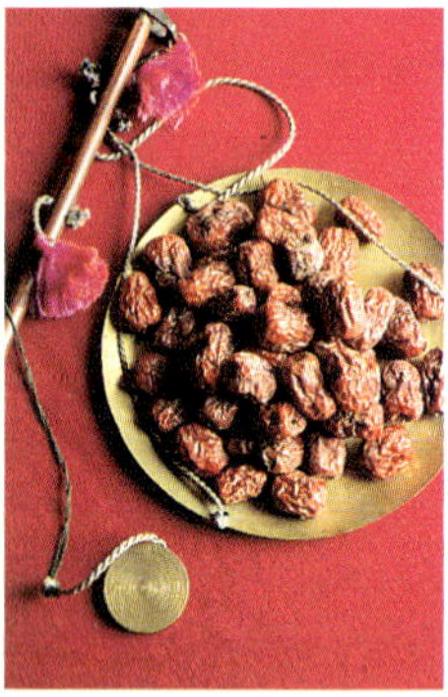

Jujube, Common

大枣

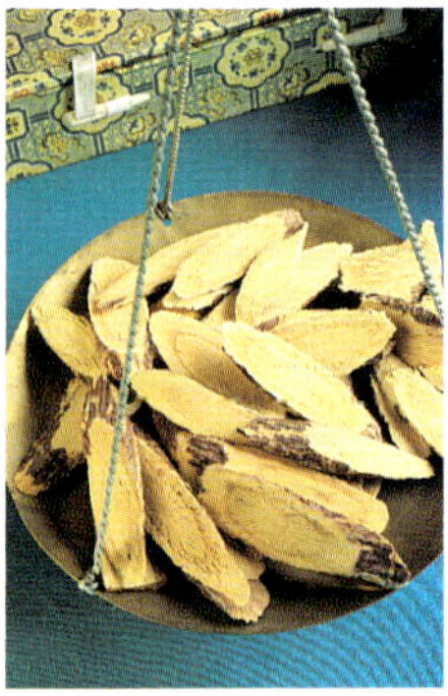

Licorice

甘草

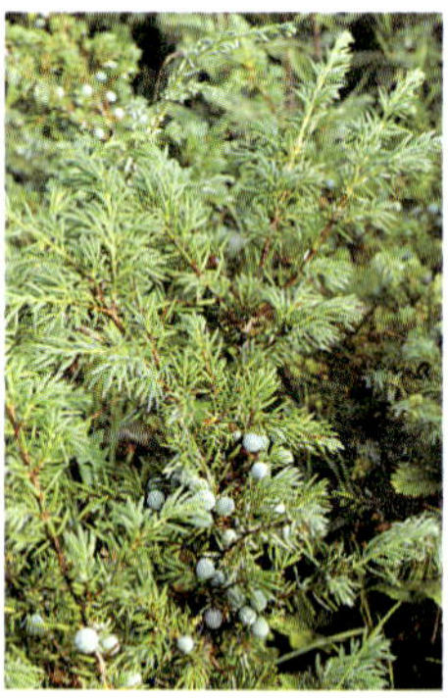

Juniper *(Juniperus communis)*

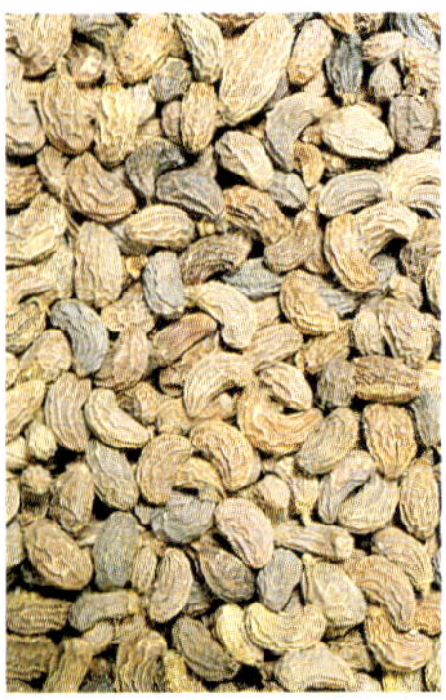

Ligustrum

女貞子

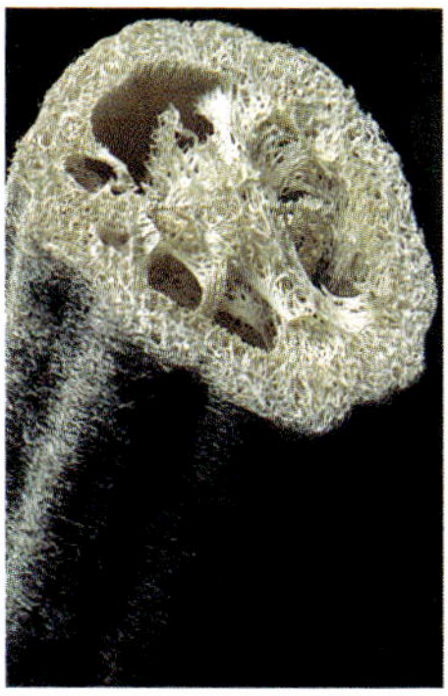

Luffa

丝瓜络

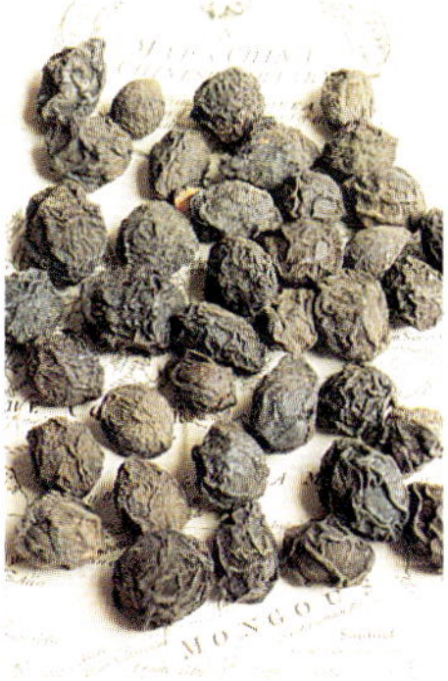

Mume

乌梅

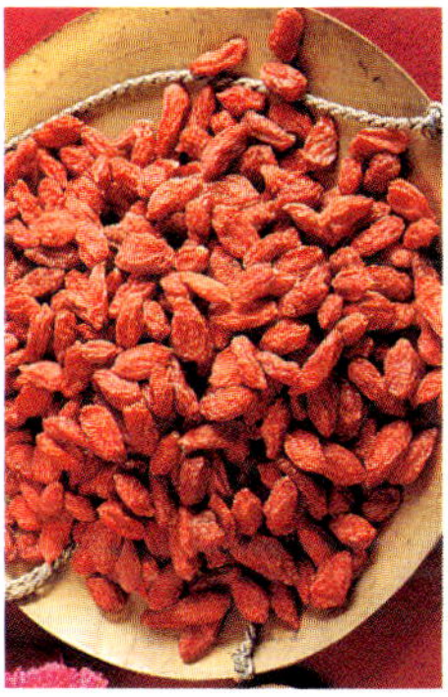

Lycium

枸杞子

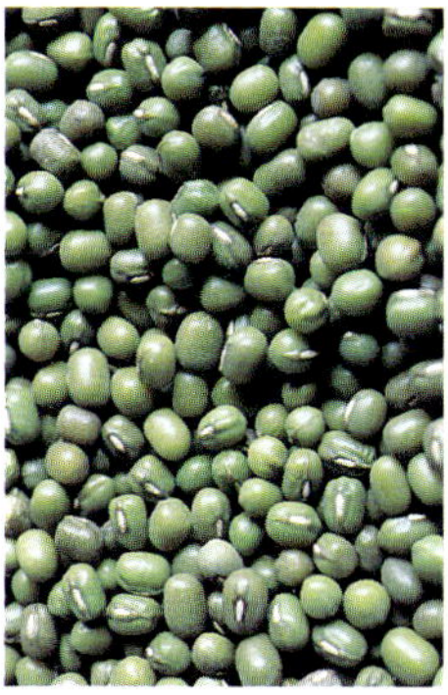

Mung bean

绿豆

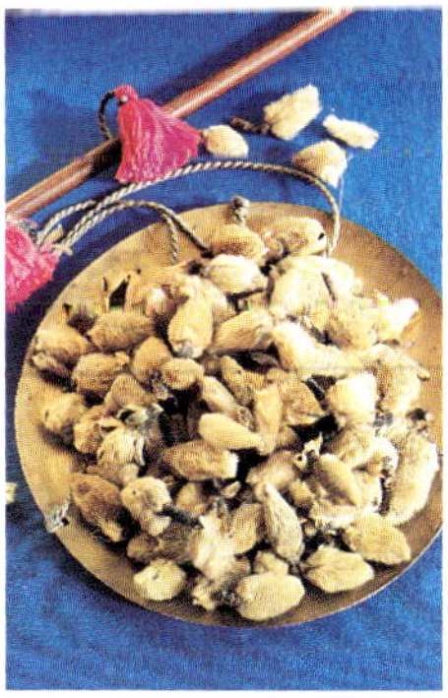

Magnolia

辛夷花

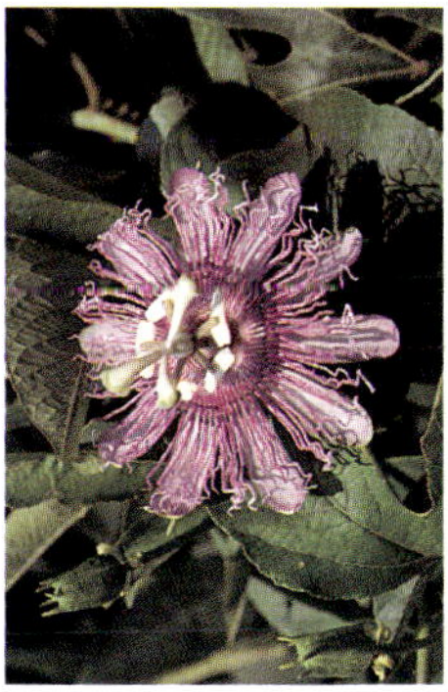

Passion flower
(Passiflora incarnata)

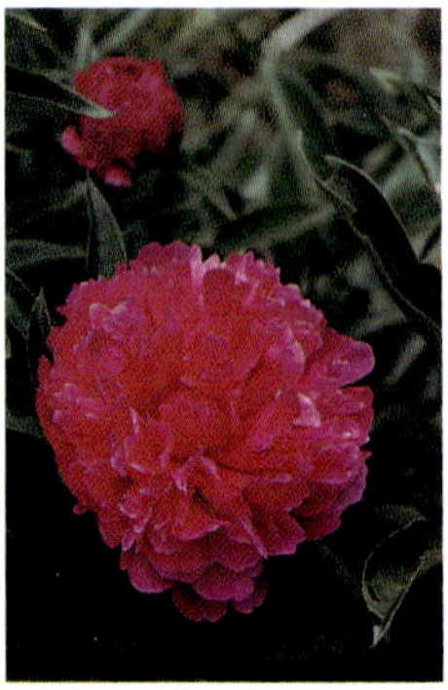

Peony, Red
(Paeonia lactiflora)

芍药

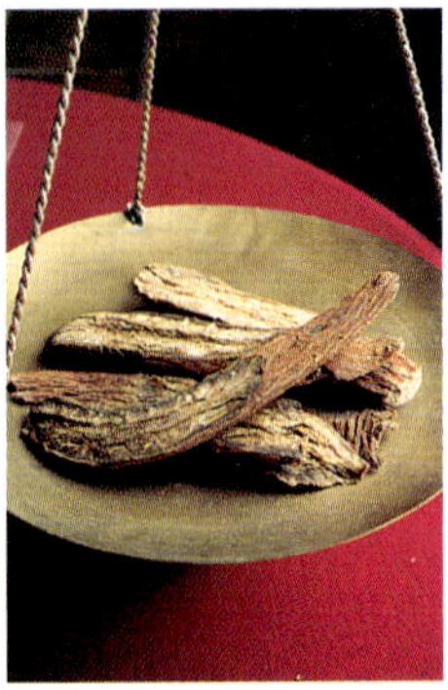

Red Sage

丹参

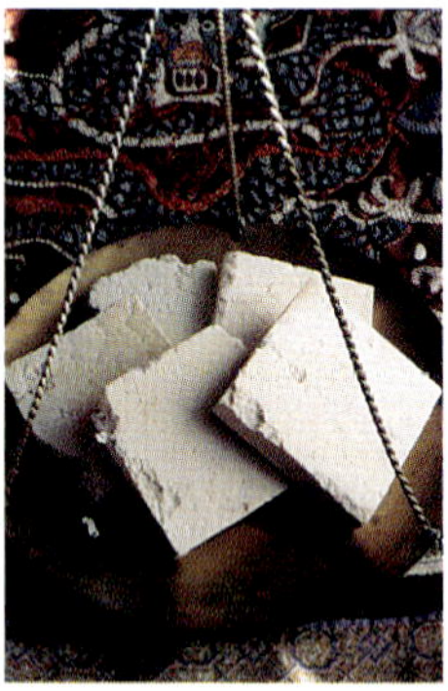

Poria

茯苓

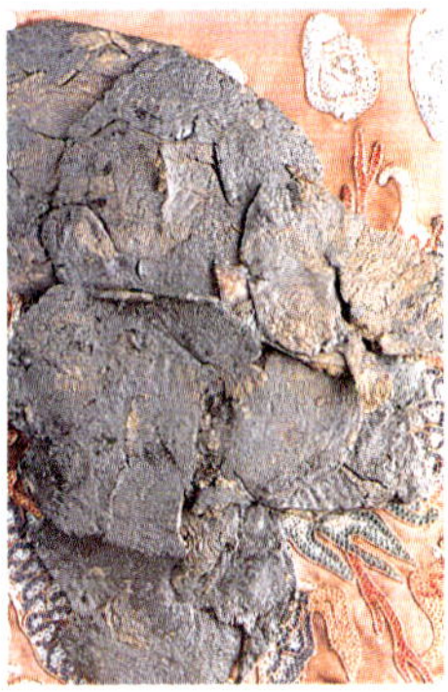

Rehmannia

地黄

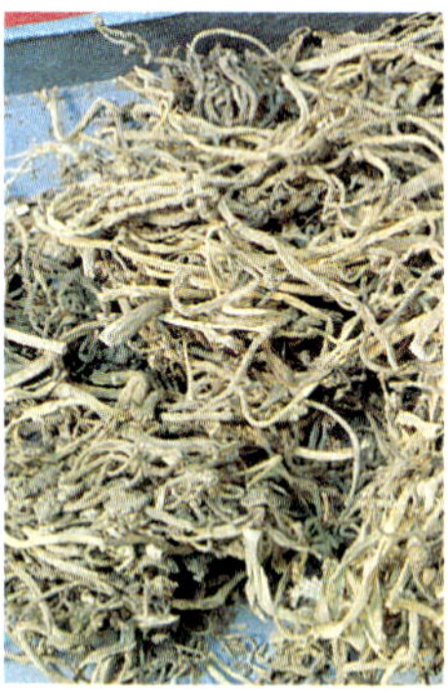

Purslane, Common

馬齿莧

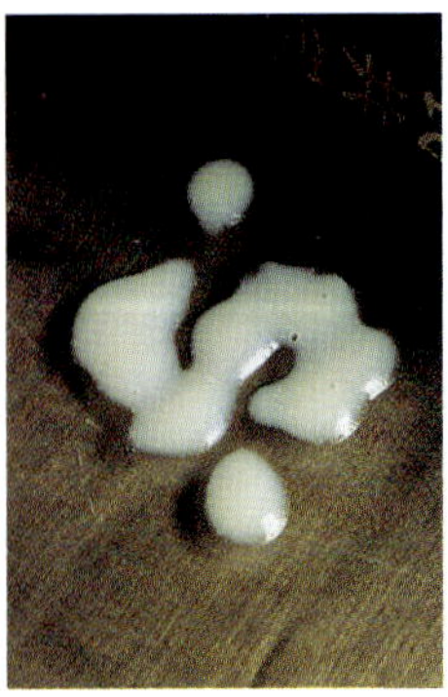

Royal Jelly

蜂乳

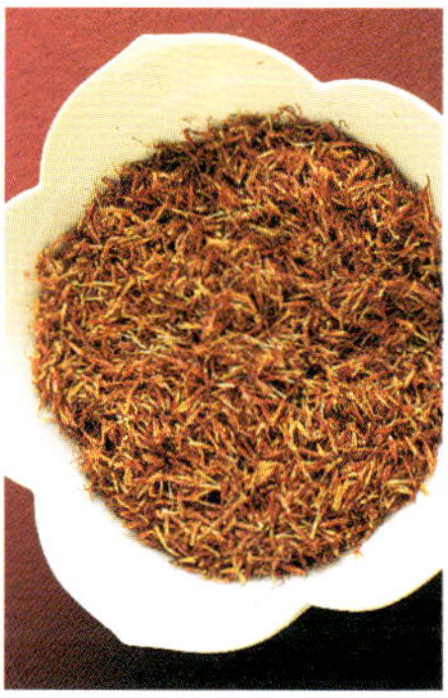

Safflower

红花

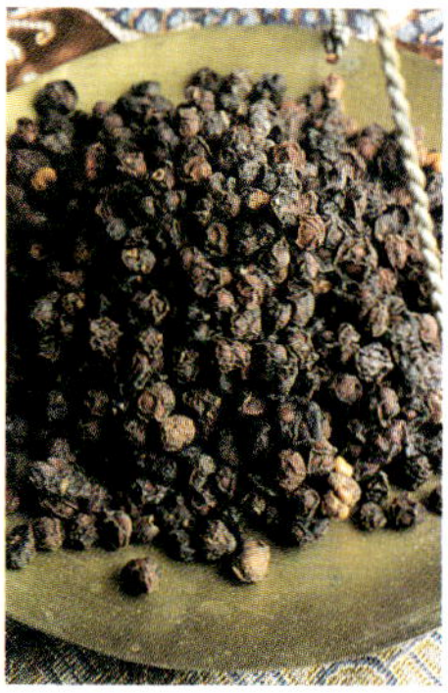

Schisandra

五味子

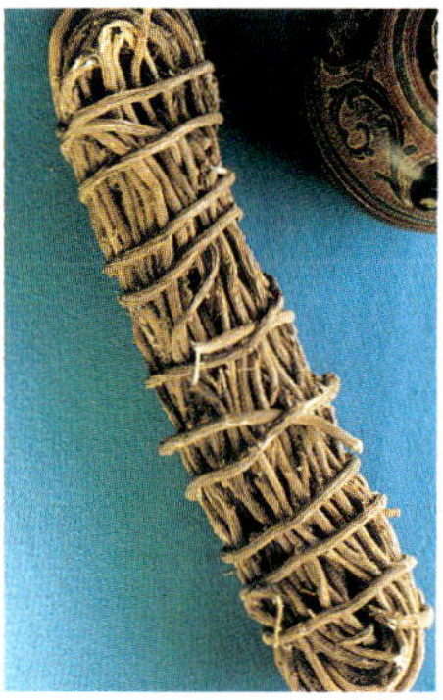

Sarsaparilla

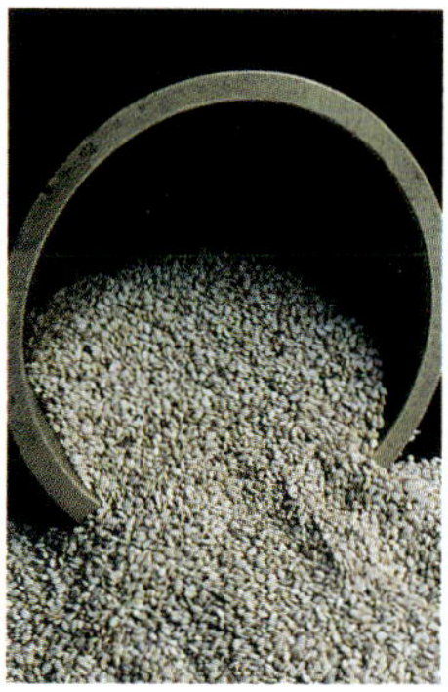

Sesame

芝麻

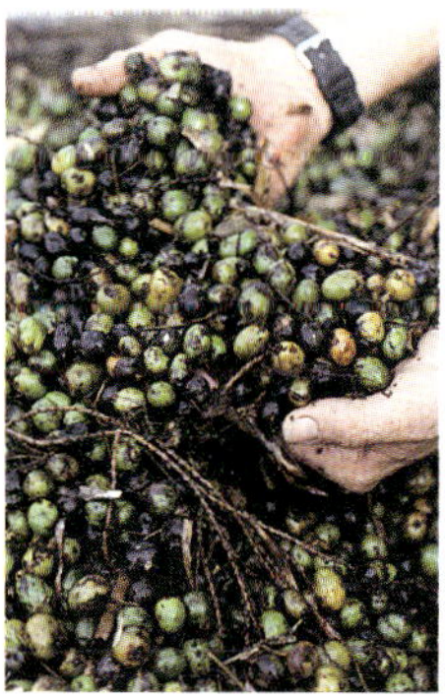

Saw Palmetto
(Serenoa repens)

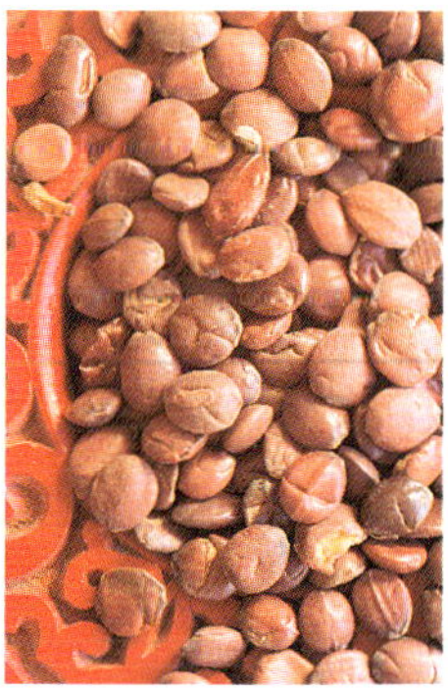

Sour Jujube Kernel

酸枣仁

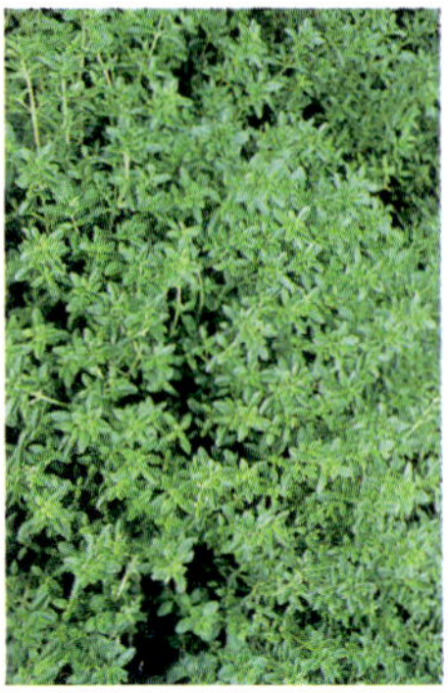

Thyme
(Thymus vulgaris)

地椒

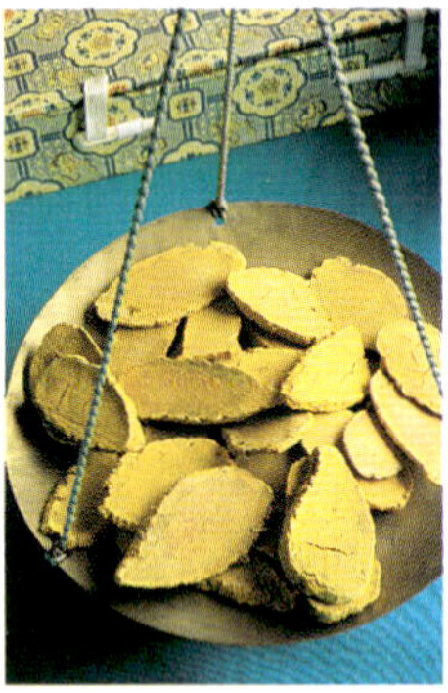

Turmeric

姜黄

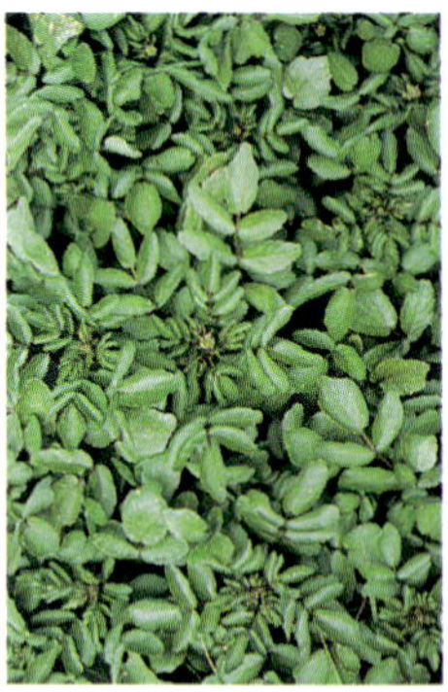

Watercress
(Nasturtium officinale)

西洋菜

GLOSSARY

Adaptogenic. Increasing the body's resistance to outside stresses of various kinds without causing it to deviate from its normal functions; normalizing body functions.
Amenorrhea. Absence or abnormal stoppage of the menses.
Analgesic. Pain relieving.
Angina pectoris. Chest pain.
Anthelmintic. Destroying or preventing infection caused by parasitic worms.
Antiallergic. Preventing or stopping allergic reactions.
Antiandrogenic. Counteracting androgenic (male hormonal) activity.
Anti-arteriosclerotic. Preventing arteriosclerosis.
Anti-atherosclerotic. Preventing atherosclerosis.
Antiestrogenic. Counteracting estrogenic activity.
Antiirritant. Relieving irritation.
Antilipemic. Preventing lipemia.
Antimutagenic. Opposing the effects of mutagens or substances that cause genetic change (mutation); mutagens include various radiations and cancer-causing chemicals.
Antioxidant. Opposing oxidative reactions promoted by oxygen or peroxides. These reactions produce free radicals as by-products, which, if not prevented or removed, may cause cell damage, leading to various illnesses, including degenerative diseases (*e.g.*, arthritis), heart diseases, and even cancer.
Antispasmodic. Preventing or relieving convulsions or spasms.
Antitussive. Suppressing or relieving cough.
Aphrodisiac. Exciting sexual desire.
Arrhythmia. Abnormal heart beat.
Astringent. Toning up.
Arteriosclerosis. A chronic disease in which arterial walls are abnormally thickened and hardened.
Atherosclerosis. A form of arteriosclerosis characterized by the deposition of fats (*e.g.*, cholesterol) in and the hardening of the inner layer of the arteries.
Bronchiospasmolytic. Relieving the abnormal contraction of the bronchi.
Calmative. Calming or sedative.
Carminative. Inducing expulsion of gas so as to relieve pain in the bowels.
Choleretic. Stimulating the production of bile by the liver.
Colic. Sharp sudden abdominal pain.
Colitis. Inflammation of the large intestine, including Crohn's disease, ulcerative colitis and irritable bowel syndrome.
Counterirritant. Agent applied locally to produce superficial inflammation with the object of reducing inflammation in deeper adjacent tissues.

Decoction. Chinese medicines are usually taken in the form of a water extract. This extract is prepared by boiling the herbs in water slowly for between half an hour to several hours in an earthen or porcelain pot. Traditionally, pots made of metal (especially iron) are not used. To prepare the extract (called decoction), the herb is placed in the pot and covered completely with water plus another one-third to half as much. The mixture is boiled, usually gently, until about one-third of the liquid remains. The liquid is then decanted off. Another smaller portion of water is added to the partially extracted herb and boiled once more down to about one-third or one-quarter of the volume. This second extract is decanted off and added to the first to form the complete decoction.
The main purpose of boiling (decocting) is to extract the active ingredients and, in the case of herbal combinations (formulas), also to produce active compounds through the interaction of different herbs. Another purpose is to render the toxic herbs less toxic and thus safer to use.
Demulcent. Soothing or protecting inflamed or abraded mucous surfaces.
Detoxifier (detoxicant). An agent that removes or speeds up the removal of toxins from the body.
Diaphoretic. Increasing perspiration.
Diuretic. Increasing the flow of urine.
Dysmenorrhea. Menstrual pain.
Dysuria. Painful or difficult urination.
Eczema. An itching skin inflammation with crusted lesions.
Edema. Excessive accumulation of fluid in the tissues.
Emmenagogue. Agent that promotes menstrual flow.
Emollient. Softening tissues, especially the skin and mucous membranes.
Enteritis. Inflammation of the bowels, especially the small intestine, caused by bacteria, viruses or some functional disorders.
Erysipelas. A contagious skin infection caused by a bacterium (*Streptococcus* sp.).
Estrogenic. Female hormonal.
Expectorant. Promoting the discharge or expulsion of mucus from the nose or throat.
Extract. Solution (as of water or alcohol) of essential constituents of a plant or other material.
Febrifuge. Reducing body temperature.
Flatulence. Excess of air or gas in the stomach and intestines.
Furuncle. Boil; a bacterial skin infection.
Hemostatic. Stopping the flow of blood.
Hypercholesterolemia (hypercholesteremia). Excess of cholesterol in the blood.
Hyperlipemia (hyperlipidemia). Excess of lipids or fats in the blood.
Hypertension. High blood pressure.
Hypertensive. Raising blood pressure.
Hypoglycemic. Lowering blood sugar.

Hypolipemic. Lowering blood lipids.
Hypotensive. Lowering blood pressure.
Immunomodulating. Balancing the immune system.
Immunopotentiating. Stimulating the immune system.
Immunostimulant. Stimulating the immune system.
Leukopenia (leukocytopenia). Abnormal decrease of while blood cells (leukocytes).
Leukorrhea. A clear or pearly-white vaginal discharge.
Leukorrhagia. Profuse leukorrhea.
Lipemia (lipidemia). Hyperlipemia.
Lumbago. Pain in the lower back.
Mastitis. Breast inflammation.
Menorrhalgia. Distress associated with menstruation, including premenstrual tension and menstrual pain.
Metrorrhagia. Abnormal uterine bleeding.
Neuralgia. Acute pain that follows the course of a nerve.
Neurasthenia. A condition of nervous exhaustion and physical tiredness that often follows depression.
Neurodermatitis. An itching skin disorder of anxious and nervous individuals, with scratches and skin thickening present on exposed areas of the body, including the forearms and forehead.
Palpitation. Pounding or racing of the heart.
Pruritus. Itching.
Purpura. A group of disorders characterized by purplish or brownish red discoloration, easily visible through the skin, caused by hemorrhage in the tissues (e.g., black and blue marks, bruises).
Pyogenic. Pus-forming.
***Qi* (*chi*)**. Traditional Chinese medical term with no English or modern medical equivalent; the closest modern equivalent includes "energy," "vital energy," and "functional activities."
Rhinitis. Inflammation of the mucous membranes of the nose.
Rubefacient. Applied externally to irritate or produce redness of the skin.
Scleroderma. Chronic hardening and shrinking of the connective tissue of any part of the body, including the skin, heart, esophagus, kidney and lung.
Scrofula. Used here for inflammation of the lymph nodes.
Sinusitis. Inflammation of a sinus, for example nasal sinuses, causing congestion and blockage.
Spermatorrhea. Involuntary, too frequent, and excessive discharge of semen without copulation.
Stomachic. Stimulating the stomach.
Tinnitus. A noise (*e.g.*, ringing) in the ears.
Tonic. Stimulating, invigorating, or increasing body tone and building up strength and resistance.
Urticaria. Hives.
Vasodilating. Dilating the blood vessels.

Index

abdominal distension, herbs for treating, 10, 40
abdominal mass, herbs for treating, 74,88
abdominal pain, herbs for treating, 9,26,45, 56, 69,74
abortion, herb for preventing, 22
abscess, herbs for treating, 5,16,56,72
acetylenes, occurrence, 7
acne, herbs for treating, 66,67,71,74
acne cream, 31,69
aconite poisoning, herb for treating, 66
adaptogenic, 24,83
adenine, 16,71
adenosine: occurrence, 33,34,49; biological effects, 33,34
adenosine-3',5'-monophosphate. *See* cyclic AMP
AIDS, herbs for treating, 5
alcoholism, herbs for treating, 1,9. *See* also drunkenness and hangover
alfalfa, 1
alkaloids: occurrence, 18,34,64,85; biological effects, 64, 86
allergies, herbs for treating, 30,31,63,65
allergies, substances that cause, xv,xvi,9,16, 37
Allium sativum, 35
Aloe barbadensis, 2
aloe vera, 2,3
aloe vera, adulteration of, xi,2,22
amenorrhea, herbs for treating, 9,21,45,59, 74,78
amino acids, 6,9,16,18,26,33,37, 49,51,60,75,76
anabolic, 34
anabolic supplements, 80
analgesic, 2,12,26,34,37,38,40,44,59,69,70,74, 78,80,88
anemia, herbs for treating, 18,21,51,84,90
anesthetic, local. *See* local anesthetic
angelica, 4
Angelica archangelica, 4
Angelica sinensis, 21
angelica, Chinese, 21
angina pectoris, herbs for treating, 16,54,74
angiosarcoma, herb for treating, 48
anthelmintic, 35,45,87. *See* also parasites
Anthemis nobilis, 37
anthraglycosides, occurrence and biological effects, 3
anti-aging herbs, 28,44,60,61,71
anti-allergic, 30,34,56,58,63,65. *See* also allergies
antiandrogenic, 81
antiarthritic. *See* arthritis
antiasthmatic, 34. *See* also asthma
anti-atherosclerotic, 14,28,58,74
antibacterial, 11,15,16,19,28,30,34,35,38,44,47,63,69,72,74, 77,87
anticholinergic, 34
anticoagulant, 7,34,74,78
anticonvulsive, 34
antidiarrheal, 14,45,54
antidiuretic, 14
antiemetic, 40
antiestrogenic, 81
antifungal, 11,16,19,63,69,72,87
antihistaminic, 49,63,65
anti-infective, 37
antiinflammatory, 2,5,7,12,13,16,17,19,24,28,30,34,37,40,44, 46, herb for treating 47,49,56,58,59,63,64, 69,70,72,74,77, 80,81,88
anti-irritant, 46
antilipemic. *See* hypolipemic
antimicrobial, 32,37,38,44,63,65,69,70. *See* also antibacterial, antifungal and antiviral
antimutagenic, 14,58,61,70,71,77,83,88
antinausea, 40
antioxidants, conventional, 72
antioxidant, xix,1,5,13,14,24,26,28,30,34,38,46,49,53, 56,57,60-62,74,83,87,88
antipyretic. See febrifuge
antirheumatic. *See* rheumatism
antiseptic, 53,87
antispasmodic, 35,37,45,68,70,87,88
antistress, 18,24,42
antitumor, 7,19,24,34,48,58,70,71,74,75,77,88
antitussive, 34,38,56
antiviral, 5,11,14,16,19,28,30,38,47,48,63,69
aphrodisiac, 26,35,44
Apiaceae, 4,13,21,44
Apidae, 77
Apis mellifera, 77
Apium graveolens, 13
appendicitis, acute, herbs for treating, 38,49, 72
appetite, lack of, herbs for treating, 5,10,15, 18,19,33, 42,51,87
appetite stimulant, 1,12,15,40,45,71,88
Araliaceae, 24,42
arrhythmia, herb for treating, 33
arrowroot starch, 54
arsenic poisoning. *See* poisoning, heavy metal
arteriosclerosis, herbs for treating, 35,36,45
arthritic pain, herbs for relieving, 10,21,59,80
arthritis, herbs for treating, 1,4,11-13,24,38,75,77, 84
aspartame, toxicities of, xvi,37,76
aspirin, 47
Asteraceae, 7,10,15,16,19,37,78
asthma, herbs for treating, 18,33,34,65,81,83
astragalus, 5-8,10,18,51,77
Astragalus membranaceus, 5
astringent, 9,38,65,69,83
athlete's foot, cosmetics for, 31
atractylodes, 7,10
Atractylodes spp., 7,10
backache, herbs for treating, 24,28,58,60,75. *See* also lumbago
bacterial infections. *See* infections, bacterial
bad breath, herbs for treating, 55. *See* also "hot" and "toxic" conditions
baizhu, 7,8,10
barley, as adulterant, 49,50
bath preparations, 78
"beautifying" herbs, 58,61
bed wetting, herb for treating, 14
bedsores, herb for treating, 60
bee pollen, 9
benign prostatic hyperplasia. *See* BPH
benzene poisoning. *See* poisoning, benzene
bergapten, occurrence and toxicity, 4
beriberi, herb for treating, 26
berberine, 31
betaine, 34
β-bisabolol, occurrence and biological effects,37
bites, insect, herbs for treating, 2,72,84
bites, poisonous snake, herb for treating, 12
bitters, alcoholic, 53
bitter principles, occurrence, 15,19
blackheads, 66,67
bladder infections, herb for treating, 53

bladder stone, herb for treating, 1
bleeding. *See* specific types, e.g., nosebleed, vomiting blood, etc.
bleeding and swollen gums, herb for treating, 37
blood abnormalities, herb-induced, 1
blood-activating properties, 69,74
blood circulation, herbs that promote, 21,59, 74
blood-cooling properties, 72,75
blood-deficiency conditions, herbs for treating, 18,69
blood formation. *See* hematopoiesis
blood-invigorating properties, 78
blood-nourishing properties, 58,69
blood-purifying properties, 21,80
blood stasis, herbs that break up, 9,24,69,74, 78,88
blood tonic. *See* tonic, blood
bloodshot eyes. *See* eyes, red or bloodshot
bloody stool, herb for treating, 72
bloody urine, herbs for treating, 35,88
body fluids, herbs to promote secretion of, 51,54,65, 85
body functions, herb that normalizes 51
BPH, herb for treating, 81
brain tonic. *See* tonic, brain
Brassica campestris, 9
breast, underdeveloped, herb for treating, 81
breast problems (inflammation, lumps, etc.), herbs for treating,19. *See* also milk flow, lack of
bronchial problems, herbs for treating, 4,56, 87
bronchiospasmolytic, 87
bronchitis, chronic, herbs for treating, 19,33,35, 81
bronchitis, herbs for treating, 13,26,87
bruises, herbs for treating, 19,87,88
buckwheat, 9,38
burns, herbs for treating, 2,38,40,44,60,66,67, 72,84
caffeic acid, 87
caffeine, 44
calmative, 13,33,37,71,74. *See* also sedative
Campanulaceae, 18
cancer, herbs for treating, 8,48,65,68,81
canker sores. *See* mouth ulcers
cangzhu, 7,10,11
Caprifoliaceae, 47
capsaicin, occurrence and biological effects, 12
capsicum, 12
Capsicum spp., 12
carbohydrates. *See* polysaccharides
carbuncle, herbs for treating, 19,28,66,70,84
carcinogens, substances to prevent formation of, 48
cardiotonic, 15,45,58,76,78
cardiovascular effects, 74,78
cardiovascular problems, herbs for treating, 74, 78
carminative, 4,12,35,37,40,53,80,87
β-carotene: occurrence, 12,24,51,60,72; biological effects, 60
carotenoids: occurrence and biological effects, 14,20
carrot, 20
Carthamus tinctorius, 78
carvacrol, 87
cassava poisoning. *See* poisoning, cassava
catechins, occurrence and biological effects, 14, 53
cayenne pepper, 12
celery seed (fruit), 13
Centella asiatica, 44
chalcones, occurrence and biological effects, 78
chamazulene, occurrence and biological effects, 37
chamomile, English or Roman, allergies to, 37
chamomile, German. *See* German chamomile
chapped lips, herb for treating, 26
chemotherapy toxic effects, herbs for treating, 7,8,58,60, 68
Cherokee rosehip, 14
chest, tightness in, herbs for treating, 69,74
chest, tightness in, soup for, 85
chest pain, herbs for treating, 59,78,88
chicory, 15
chilblain, herb for treating, 12. *See* also frostbite
chili pepper, 12
Chinese cinnamon, 70
Chinese foxglove, 75,76
Chinese pearl barley, 49,50
Chinese rosehip, 14
chlorogenic acid, occurrence and biological effects, 48
cholagogue, 15,35. *See* also choleretic
choleretic, 19,88
cholesterol absorption, herb that prevents, 1
choline, occurrence, 15,16,37,71
chrysanthemum, 16,17,55
Chrysanthemum, 15
Cichorium intybus, 15
cinchona bark, 31
ciwujia, 24
cleansers, cosmetic, 38,59
cleansing properties, 2
codonopsis, 18
Codonopsis pilosula, 18
coffee, 48
coffee flavor enhancer, 15,19
coix seed, 49
Coix lachryma-jobi, 49
coixans, occurrence and biological effects, 49
coixol, occurrence and biological effects, 49
Cola nitida,44
cold-natured herbs, 69
cold limbs, herb for treating, 42
colds, herbs for treating, 4,5,10,11,16,30,31,35,40,44,47,54, 63,80,81
colic, herbs for treating, 12,37,45,53,88
colitis, herb for treating, 72. *See* also diarrhea
collagen, herb that promotes synthesis of, 62
colorant, natural, 79,88
complexion, herbs to benefit or improve,33,51,60,61, 69
conjunctivitis, herb for treating, 16
constipation, herbs for treating, 7,9,19,21,28, 84
constipation, habitual in the elderly, herb for treating, 50
cooling herbs, 26,42
Coptis species, 31
coronary heart disease, herbs for treating, 33,36,74,78
cosmetics, adverse effects, 64
cosmetics, 3,8,17,31,38,46,57,58,62,65,67,69, 71,77,79,84
cough, herbs for treating, 4,18,35,38,40,56,60, 71,81,83
cough, chronic, herbs for treating, 14,26,33,65
cough, dry, herb for treating, 91
cough, whooping, herbs for treating, 35,87
coughing blood, herb for treating, 9
coumarins: occurrence, 1,4,37,72; phototoxicity of, 4
coumarin glycosides, occurrence, 13,15,24
counter-irritant, 12
cramps, herbs for treating, 12,21. *See* also menstruation difficulties
crataegolic acid, occurrence and biological effects, 46
Crataegus spp., 45
creams, cosmetic, 17,38
Cruciferae, 90
Cucurbitaceae, 59

Cupressaceae, 53
cure-all, 35
Curcuma longa, 88
Curcuma domestica, 88
curcumin, occurrence and biological effects, 88
curry, 26,88
cyclic AMP, occurrence and biological effects, 51,85
cyclic GMP, 85
cystitis, chronic, herb for treating, 81
dandelion, 19,20
dandruff, herb for treating, 35
dandruff, shampoo for, 31
danggui, 4,21,22
danggui, caution in pregnancy, 22
danggui, European. *See* lovage
dangshen, 18
danshen, 74
danshensu, occurrence and biological effects, 74
daucosterol, 75
dazao, 51
degenerative diseases, treatment of 11
demulcent, 26,56
depression, herb that alleviates, 10
dermatitis, herb for treating, 72
dermatitis, contact, herbs for treating, 45,46
dermatitis, herb-induced, 4
detoxicant, 2,16,17,19,28,30,32,38,40,44,47,51,54,56,59,66, 69,72,80,83,90,91
diabetes, herbs for treating, 1,5,18,54,60,65, 72,75,77
diaphoretic, 4,37,40,54,68,80,87
diarrhea, herbs to treat, 5,7,9,10,12,35,40,45,49,51,54,71,87
diarrhea, chronic, herbs for treating, 14,18,65, 83. *See* also enteritis and colitis
diet soda, adverse effects, 76
Dietary Supplement Health and Education Act of 1994 (DSHEA), xvii
digestive aid, 12,13,14,15,16,19,26,35,40,45, 53
digitalis, 76
dihuang, 75
diphtheria, herb for treating, 35
disinfectant, herbal, 10, 11, 38
diterpernoids, occurrence and biological effects, 74
diuretic, 1,4,5,7,9,10,13,15,19,24,34,35,44,49,53,58,66,71, 72,75,80,81,90
dizziness, herbs for treating, 16,28,58,60,69, 84
dong quai, 21
dopa, 72
dopamine, 72
drug development, 89
drug poisoning. *See* poisoning, drug
drug use, excessive, iv
drunkenness, herb for treating, 54
dry skin, herb for treating, 51
duodenal ulcer, herbs for treating, 40,56. *See* also peptic ulcer
dysentery, herbs for treating, 35,40,47,66,72
dysmenorrhea, herb for treating, 9
dyspepsia. *See* indigestion
dysuria, herbs for treating, 9,30,55,71,72,90, 91
earache, herbs for treating, 35,72
eczema, herbs for treating, 9,10,16,19,49,65,72,74,75, 90
edema, herbs for reducing, 5,10,24,49,71,88
eleuthero, 24,25
Eleutherococcus senticosus, 24
eleutherosides, 24. *See* also glycosides
"elixir of life," 33
emmenagogic, 4,13
emollient, 2,26
energy, lack of, herb for treating, 60
energy flow, herbs that promote, 59,88
"energy" formulas, composition of, 18,77
"energy" tonic. *See* tonic, *qi*
enteritis, herbs for treating, 14,45,47,49,66,72. *See* also diarrhea
EPA (Environmental Protection Agency), 38, 39
en-yn-dicycloether, occurrence and biological effects,37
Ephedra species,31
ephedrine, 31
epidemic, practice during, 10
epilepsy, herb for treating, 68
erysipelas, herbs for treating, 30,66
estrogenic, 24,81
eucalyptus, 63
"evil"or"evil wind"intraditional Chinese medicine,10,31
expectorant, 4,26,35,38,56,81,87,90
eyes, excessive tearing of, herb for treating, 16
eyes, red or bloodshot, herbs for treating, 16,55, 90,91. See also "hot" and "toxic" conditions
facial dark spots, cosmetics for, 8,71
facial dark spots, herbs for removing, 58,63, 90
facial scrubs, 59
facial treatment formulas of Chinese imperial courts, 71
Fagopyrum esculentum, 9
false saffron, 78
fatigue, herbs for relieving, 5,10,18,34,42,38, 51,70. *See* also neurasthenia
fatty acids, occurrence and biological effects, 33,44, 53,58,72,78,85. *See* also omega-3 acids
FDA (Food and Drug Administration), x,xvi, xvii, 37, 68,76,81
febrifuge, 16,18,19,26,30,35,42,44,47,49,54,59,74,76, 80
female problems, herb for treating, 14. *See* also menstruation difficulties
fenugreek, 26,27
fenugreek, caution in pregnancy, 26,27
fetus-calming properties, 7,22,75,79
fever, herbs for treating. See febrifuge
fever-reducing properties. *See* febrifuge
"feverish air" conditions. *See* "hot" and "toxic" conditions
"five-flavored seed." *See wuweizi*
flatulence, herbs for treating, 4,7,12,19,53,80, 88
flavonoids: occurrence, 1,4,5,6,9,13,14,16,26,30,37,44, 46,48,51,53,57,64,72,78,85,87; biological effects, xiii xiv,1,5, 14, 26,46,57,64, 85,86
flavonoid glycosides. *See* flavonoids
flu, herbs for treating, 5,11,16,30,31,47,54
fluid retention: due to herbs, 56; herbs to treat, 1,7
food flavoring, 56
food poisoning. *See* poisoning, food
forgetfulness, herbs for treating, 71,85
forsythia, 30
Forsythia suspensa, 30
forsythol, 30
fo-ti, 7,28,38
fo-ti, cured and raw, 28
freckles. *See* facial dark spots
frostbite, herbs for treating, 12,45,60
fructose, potential source of, 15
fuling, 71
fuling breads and cakes, 71
fumigation. *See* operating rooms

furuncles, herbs for treating, 19,26,60
gallstones, herbs for treating, 15,19. *See* also bladderstone
ganoderma, 33,34
Ganoderma spp., 33
garlic, 35,36
gastritis, chronic, herb for treating, 87
gastroenteritis, herb for treating, 37
gegen, 54
German chamomile, 37
germanium, 34
giant knotweed, 38,39
gin, ingredients in, 53
ginger, 40,41,70
ginseng, 7,10,22,24,33,34,42,43
ginseng, adulteration, xi
ginseng, American and Asian, 42,43,77,83
ginseng, poor man's. *See* poor man's ginseng
ginseng, Siberian. *See* eleuthero
"ginseng abuse syndrome," x
ginseng leaf, Asian, properties of, 43
ginseng saponins. *See* ginsenosides and panaxosides
ginsenosides, occurrence and biological effects, 24,43
glands, swollen. *See* swollen glands
glutathione, occurrence and biological effects, 72
glycolipids, 49
glycosides, occurrence and biological effects, xiii,24,58, 75,76. *See* also saponins
Glycyrrhiza spp., 56
glycyrrhizin, adverse effects, 56
gonadotropic, 24
gonorrhea, herb for treating, 80
gotu-kola, 44
gout, herbs for treating, 13,19,26,35,37,80,90
Gramineae, 49
green gram, 66
gums, swollen. *See* swollen gums
hair, premature graying of, herbs to treat,28,58,75, 84
hair-growth liniments, 31,78. See also tonic, hair
hair loss, herbs for treating, 28,84
hair tonic. *See* tonic, hair
hangover, herb for treating, 43,55
hawthorn, Chinese and Western (English and European), 45,46
hay fever, herbs for treating, 30,63,64,65. *See* also allergies
10-HDA, occurrence and biological effects, 77
head, heaviness of, herbs for treating, 55. See also "hot" and "toxic" conditions
headache, herbs for treating, 16,21,35,54,55, 63,69,72
headache, nervous, herb for treating, 68
healing. *See* wound-healing
heart problems, herbs for treating, 33,42,45, 78
heart tonic. *See* cardiotonic
heat-dispersing properties, 30,49,66,72,75,90, 91
heat rash, herb for treating, 66
heatstroke, herb for treating, 66. *See* also sunstroke
hematemesis. *See* vomiting blood
hematoma, herb for treating, 12
hematopoiesis, herbs that promote, 21,75
hemoglobin, herb that raises level of, 60
hemorrhoids, herbs for treating, 40,59,72,84
hemostatic, 1,9,72,75
hepatitis, herbs to treat, 15,16,19,33,35,38,44,48,74,77, 83
herb, definition of, i
herb processing, 28,75
herb safety and toxicity, xv,xvi
herbal combinations, rationale of, xv,68
herbal formulas, 56
herbs, how they work, xiii
hernia, herbs for treating, 26,40
heshouwu, 28
high blood pressure. *See* hypertension
honeybee, 77
honeysuckle, 47,48
honghua, 78
hongzao, 51
hookworm infection, herbs for treating, 65,87. *See* also anthelmintic
hormonal "messenger," 51
"hot" conditions. *See* "hot" and "toxic" conditions
"hot" and "toxic" conditions, herbs for treating, 19,26,30,31, 47,55,66,69,90,91
"hot" and "toxic" conditions, symptoms, 55, 91
hot pepper, 12
huanglian, 31
huangqi, 5
huo xue hua yu (activating blood circulation to disperse stasis) herbs, 74,78
huzhang, 38
hydroxyproline, herb that increases level of, 62
10-hydroxy-*trans*-2-decenoic acid. *See* 10-HDA
hypercholesterolemic, 34
hyperglycemic, 18
hyperlipemia, herbs for treating, 28,33,36,45
hypersensitive dentin, herb for treating, 35
hypertension, herb-induced, 56
hypertension, herbs for treating, 14,16,18,21, 33,35,36,45,51, 54,74,77
hypertensive, 72
hypnotic formulas, 85
hypocholesterolemic, 88
hypoglycemic, 7,19,24,26,34,42,49,58,61
hypolipemic, 14,28,34,58,61,66,78
hypotensive, 5,13,16,18,24,30,34,35,42,45,61, 75,78,88. *See* also cardiovascular effects
hysteria, herbs for treating, 35,51,68
immunomodulating effects, 5,18,24,34,42,46,58,60,70, 71,75
immunopotentiating effects, 7,18,28,61,77,78
immunosuppressive effects, 78
impotence, herbs for treating, 24,26,42,83
indigestion, herbs to treat, 4,7,10,15,19, 33,37,45,66, 90
infantile convulsions, herb for treating, 37
infections, bacterial, herbs for treating, 19,30,36,37,47, 55. *See* also antibacterial
infections, fungal, herb for treating, 36. *See* also antifungal
infections, viral, herbs for treating, 10,19,30, 31,47,55. *See* also antiviral
inflammations, herbs for treating. *See* antiinflammatory
inflammation of lymph nodes. *See* scrofula
inflammatory kidney diseases, contraindication in, 53
influenza. *See* flu
insects, 11,16
insect bites and stings. *See* bites
insecticidal, 88
insomnia, herbs to treat, 4,16,21,28,33,37,42,56,68,71,74,83, 85
internal organs, herb that vitalizes, 84
intybin. *See* bitter principles
inulin, occurrence, 15,18,19
iridoid glycosides, 75
irregular menses. *See* menstruation difficulties
irritability, herb for treating, 66

irritant, gastrointestinal, 53
isochlorogenic acid, 48
itching. *See* pruritus
jaundice, herbs for treating, 15,19,38,44
jinyingzi, 14
Job's tear, 49,50
joints. *See* painful joints and stiff joints
juhua, 16
jujube, Chinese, or common, 18,51,52,58,65,87
jujube, sour. *See* sour jujube kernel
jujubosides A and B, occurrence and biological effects, 86
juniper, 53
Juniperus communis, 53
kidney problems, herb for treating, 26
Kidney tonic, 28,83,84
Kidney-invigorating properties, 58,71
Kidney-nourishing properties, 60
knee pain, herbs for treating, 28,58,60
kola nut, 44
kudzu, 54,55
Labiatae, 74,87
labiatic acid, occurrence and biological effects, 87
lacquer sores, herbs for treating, 45,46. *See* also dermatitis, contact
lactucin. *See* bitter principles
laryngitis, acute, herbs for treating, 47,87. *See* also infections
laxative, 3,15,19,21,28,56,84
lead poisoning. *See* poisoning, heavy metal
learning, herb that improves, 5
lecithins, 71
Leguminosae, 1,5,26,54,56,66
leprosy, herb for treating, 44
leucoanthocyanidins, occurrence and biological effects, 14
leukemia, herb for treating, 18
leukocytopenia. *See* leukopenia
leukopenia, herb for treating, 33
leukopenia, due to chemotherapy and radiotherapy, herbs for treating, 7,58
leukorrhagia, herb for treating, 74
leukorrhea, herb for treating, 14
Li Shi-Zhen, 45,58
lianqiao, 30
licorice Chinese and European, 5,8,40,56,57,65
licorice extracts, deglycyrrhizinated, 56,57
lignans, occurrence and biological effects, xiii,xiv,24, 64,78, 83
ligustrum, 52,58,87
Ligustrum lucidum, 58
Liliaceae, 2,35,80
lingzhi, red and purple, 33
lipid peroxides, herb that lowers level of, 60
lipids, occurrence, 9,49
liver problems, herbs for treating, 19,83,88
Liver-invigorating properties, 58
Liver-nourishing properties, 60
liver-protectant, 5,7,28,30,34,38,77,80,83
Liver tonic, 28,84
local anesthetic, 63
loganin, 48
Lonicera japonica, 47
lotions, cosmetic, 17,38
lovage, contraindication in pregnancy, 22,23
lucerne, 1
ludou, 66
luffa or luffa sponge, 59
Luffa spp., 59
lumbago, herb for treating, 37. *See* also backache
lung abscess, herb for treating, 49
lung-soothing properties, 90
lycium, 60-62
Lycium spp., 60
magnolia, 63,64,70
Magnolia spp., 63
Magnoliaceae, 63
mahuang, 31
malaria, herb for treating, 40
male sexual problems, herbs to treat, 14, 26,60,81,83
male tonic. *See* tonic, male
malnutrition in children, treatment of, 77
mannentake, 33
mannitol, 58
massage preparations, 38,78
mastitis, herbs for treating, 47,48,72. *See* also breast problems
Matricaria recutita, 37
measles, herb for treating, 75
measles, herb that accelerates eruption of, 54. *See* also skin eruptions
Medicago sativa, 1
memory, herbs that improve, 5,33,70
menorrhalgia, herb for treating, 78
menstruation, herbs that regulate, 21,69,74, 78
menstruation difficulties, herbs for treating, 4,21,22,38, 45,69,74,75,78,88
mental exhaustion. *See* neurasthenia
mercury poisoning. *See* poisoning, heavy metal
metrorrhagia, herbs for treating, 9,21,72,74. *See* also menstruation difficulties
migraine, herbs for treating, 54,81
milk flow, lack of, herbs for treating, 19,59,72,84
milk flow, herbs that promote, 19,26
milk production, rBGH in, xvi,xvii
milk thistle, 83
miltirone, occurrence and biological effects, 74
monoterpene glycosides, occurrence and biological effects, 70
motion sickness, herb for treating, 40
mouth, bitter taste in, herbs for treating, 55. *See* also "hot" and "toxic" conditions
mouth, dryness of, herbs for treating, 55. *See* also "hot" and "toxic" conditions
mouth blisters, herbs for treating, 55. See also "hot" and "toxic" conditions
mouth sores, herbs for treating, 9
mouth ulcers, herbs for treating, 26,55,90,91. See also "hot" and "toxic" conditions
mouthwashes, 87
mucilage, occurrence and biological effects, 26
mucous membrane, irritated, herb for treating, 81
mume, 52,65,87
mumps, herbs for treating, 19,47,66
mung bean, 40,55,66,67
mung bean, caution, 67
muscle relaxant, 13,22,34,49,63,72
muscle pain, herbs for treating, 21,59
muscle stimulant, 22,63
mushroom poisoning. *See* poisoning, mushroom
naphthopyrone glycosides, 75
nasal cavity, herb that clears, 63,64
nasal congestion, herbs for treating, 35,40,63
nasal decongestant, 63,64
Nasturtium officinale, 90
nausea, herb for treating, 40

neck pain, herb for treating, 54. *See* also stiff neck
neolignans, occurrence and biological effects, 64
nervine. *See* calmative
nervousness, herbs for treating, 4,13,68,71
neuralgia, herbs for treating, 21,26,68
neurasthenia, herbs for treating, 14,33,42,83,85, 87
neurodermatitis, herbs for treating, 5,65,74,75
niacinamide, 72
nicotinic acid, 60,72
night blindness, herb for treating, 10
night sweat, herbs for treating, 5,14,69,75,83, 85
nightmares, herbs for treating, 33,85
nitrosamines. *See* carcinogens
nocturnal emission. *See* spermatorrhea
l-noradrenaline, 72
nose, running, herb for treating, 63
nosebleed, herbs for treating, 9,75
numbness of limbs, herb for treating, 28
Nutrasweet. *See* aspartame
"nutriceuticals," xiv
nuzhenzi, 58
Oleaceae, 30,58
oleanolic acid, occurrence and biological effects, 30, 46,52,58,65,74,87
olives, 52
omega-3 acids, 72
operating rooms, herb for sterilizing, 10,11
oroxylin A, 18
oxygen free radicals, substances that remove,57
l-pachman, occurrence and biological effects, 71
Paeonia lactiflora, 69
Paeoniaceae, 69
paeoniflorin, occurrence and biological effects, 70
pain, arthritic. *See* arthritic pain
pain, menstrual, herb for treating, 21. *See* also menstruation difficulties
pain, rheumatic. *See* rheumatic pain
pain relieving. *See* analgesic
painful joints, herbs for treating, 5,38,49,69,74
painful urination. *See* dysuria
Palmaceae, 81
palpitations, herbs for treating, 18,74,75,85
Panax ginseng, 42
Panax quinquefolius, 42
panaxosides, occurrence and biological effects, 43
paralysis, herbs for treating, 84,87
parasites, herb for treating, 65. *See* also anthelmintic
Passiflora incarnata, 68
Passifloraceae, 68
passion flower, 68
pathogens" in traditional Chinese medicine, 10,31
Pedaliaceae, 84
peony root, red and white, 69,70
peptic ulcer, herbs for treating, 1,37,56
peptides, occurrence and biological effects, 33, 49
performance-enhancing supplements, 80
perspiration, excessive, herb that stops, 85
pesticide poisoning. *See* poisoning, pesticide
Phaseolus spp., 66
phenanthrene diketones. *See* tanshinones
phenethy alcohol glycosides, 75
phenols, 19,30,44,87
phenylpropanoid glycosides, 24
phlegm, excessive, herbs for treating, 38,40, 59
phospholipids, 49
phthalides, occurrence, 13
physical exhaustion. *See* neurasthenia
pimples. *See* acne
pine, 9
Pinus species, 9
pneumonia, herb for treating, 19
poisoning, cassava, herbs for treating, 44
poisoning, benzene, herb for treating, 58
poisoning, food or drug, herbs for treating, 40,47,56,66
poisoning, heavy metal, herbs for treating, 44,47,66,80
poisoning, mushroom, herbs for treating, 33,44, 66
poisoning, pesticide, herbs for treating, 47,66
pollen. *See* bee pollen
Polygonaceae, 28,38
polygonum, 28
Polygonum ssp., 28,38
polyps, herb for treating, 65. *See* also cancer
Polyporaceae, 33,71
polysaccharides: occurrence, 5,6,7,18,24,33,43,49,60,71,75,78; biological effects, xiii,xiv,5,34,43,49,60,61,71, 75, 78
poor man's ginseng, 18
poria, 71
Poria cocos, 71
Portulaca oleracea, 72
Portulacaceae, 72
postpartum bleeding, herb for treating, 72
potassium depletion, herb-induced, 56
pregnancy, herb use during, 22,23,26,27,53, 79
premature ejaculation, herb for treating, 26. *See* also male sexual problems
Prescriptions for Fifty-Two Diseases. See Wu Shi Er Bing Fang
proanthocyanidins, 53
proazulenes, 37
prostate enlargement, herb for treating, 81. *See* also BPH
Prunus mume, 65
pruritus, herbs for treating, 28,45,46,51,54,65, 72,88
psoriasis, herbs for treating, 54,74. *See* also skin diseases
pu er cha, 16
Pueraria spp., 54
purpura, herb for treating, 51
purslane, common, 72,73
pus-expelling properties, 49
qi tonic. *See* tonic, *qi*
queen bees, 77
quinine, 31
radioprotective, 18,42,77
radiotherapy toxic effects, herbs to treat, 7, 8,58,60
rape, 9
rBGH, FDA approval, xvi,xvii
recombinant bovine growth hormone. *See* rBGH
rectal prolapse, herb for treating, 5
red date, 51
red eyes. *See* eyes, red or bloodshot
red pepper, 12
red sage, 74,78
rehmannia, raw and cured, 75,76
Rehmannia glutinosa, 75
reishi, 33
restlessness, herbs for treating, 66,75. *See* also summer heat syndrome
Rhamnaceae, 51,85
rheumatic pain, herb for treating, 40. *See* also rheumatism
rheumatism, herbs for treating, 9,10,11,12,13,19,21,24,35,38, 42,49,59,77,80,87
rhinitis, allergic. *See* hay fever
ringworm infections, herbs for treating, 35,88
rib pain, herb for treating, 88

Rosaceae, 14,45,65
Rosa laevigata, 14
rosehip, 14
roundworm infection, herb for treating, 65. *See* also anthelmintic
royal jelly, 77
RPS-b, occurrence and biological effects, 75. *See* also polysaccharides
rubefacient, 12
sabal, 81
safflower, 78,79
safflower yellow, occurrence and biological effects,78
sage, red. *See* red sage
Salvia miltiorrhiza, 74
salvianolic acid, occurrence and biological effects, 74
salvinone, occurrence and biological effeccts, 74
saponins: occurrence, 1,14,18,24,48,80,85,86; biological effects, 14,24,48,80,86
saponin glycosides. *See* saponins
sarsaparilla, Chinese, Ecuadorian, Honduran, Jamaican and Mexican, 80
saw palmetto, 81,82
schisandra, 83
Schisandra chinensis, 83
Schisandraceae, 83
sciatica, herbs for treating, 26,37
scleroderma, herbs for treating, 44, 74
sclerotium, 71
scrofula, herbs for treating, 28,30
Scrophulariaceae, 75
secologanin, 48
sedative, 13,34,42,44,45,46,58,68,70,71,74,81, 85,87
semen, herb that replenishes, 60
Serenoa repens, 81
sesame, 84
sesame oil, cosmetic and pharmaceutical use of, 84
Sesamum indicum, 84
sesquiterpene lactones, occurrence, 7
sex vigor, herb to increase, 81
shanzha, 45
sheng dihuang, 75
Shennong Herbal, 10
shingles, herbs for treating, 21,59,72,87
shortness of breath, herbs for treating, 18
shu dihuang, 75
Siberian ginseng, 24
Sichuan peppercorn, 70
silymarin, 83
sinus problems, herbs for treating, 35,54,63
sitosterol: occurrence, 75,81; biological effects, 81
skin blemishes. *See* facial dark spots
skin diseases, herbs for treating, 4,16,19,30,37, 74
skin eruptions, herbs for treating, 28,44,75
skin irritation: due to cosmetics, 64; herbs to relieve, 2,26,64
skin boils and sores, herbs for treating, 16,19,21,26,28,38,44, 47,56,66,72,74,80,84,88
skin peeling, herb for treating, 40
skin sores, unhealed, herbs for treating, 40,65
skin stimulant, 59
skin ulcers, herbs for treating, 21,44 ,60,72,74
skin-whitening properties, 77
sleep-aid products, 68
sleep-related problems, herb for treating, 85
sleepiness, herb for treating, 10
Smilax spp., 80
smoked plum, 65
snake bites. *See* bites
SOD. *See* superoxide dismutase
sodium retention, herb-induced, 56
soft drinks with herbs, 69
Solanaceae, 12,60
soothing properties, 2
sore throat, herbs for treating, 26,40,47,56,65,81
sores, chronic, herb for treating, 5
soups and soup mixes, herbal, 5,7,14,18,21,49,50,51, 54,55,58,74,83,84,85
sour date kernel, 85
sour jujube kernel, 70,85,86
sour plum drink. *See suan mei tang*
soybean, black, 40
spermatorrhea, herbs for treating, 14,26,60,71, 75,83
spinosin, occurrence and biological effects, 85
spleen problems, herbs for treating, 15,19
Spleen deficiency, herbs for treating, 5,18
Spleen-invigorating properties, 7,10,49,71
spontaneous sweating, herbs for treating, 5,7, 69,83
sprains, herbs for treating, 12,87
stamina, herbs that increase, 5,7
stasis. *See* blood stasis
steam curing. *See* herb processing
steroids, 26,44,80. *See* also sterols
steroids, addiction to, 49
sterols: occurrence, 4,6,9,18,19,24,30,33,49,51,53,71, 75,85; biological effects, xiii,24,34
stiff neck, herb for treating, 54
stiff joints, herbs for easing, 19,33,49,69,74
stimulant, 4,24,42,90. See also muscle stimulant and uterine stimulant
stimulant, central, 18,42,83
stimulant, circulatory, 12,45,78
stimulant, gastrointestinal, 12
stimulant, heart. *See* cardiotonic
stomach problems, herb for treating, 4
stomach ulcer, herbs for treating, 5,40,56. *See* also peptic ulcer
stomachache, herbs for treating, 35,40,72
stomachic, 4,12,90
Streptococcus mutans, in tooth decay, 52
stress. *See* antistress
stroke, herb for treating, 74
suan mei tang, 65
suan zao ren, 85
sulfites, allergic reactions to, xvi,16
summer heat syndrome, herb for treating, 66
sunburn, herb for treating, 2
sunstroke, herbs for treating, 42,44
superoxide dismutase, herb to raise serum level of, 60
sweetener, natural, 56
swellings, herbs that reduce, 19,30,44,47,49,66, 87,88
swertisin, occurrence and biological effects, 85, 86
swollen glands, herb for treating, 26. *See* also scrofula
swollen gums: in "hot" and "toxic" conditions, 55,91; herbs for treating, 55,84, 90,91
syphilis, herbs for treating, 44,80
systemic lupus erythematosus, herb-induced, 1
tang kuei or *tang kwei*, 21
tangshenosides, 18
tanshinones, occurrence and biological effects, 74
tapeworm infection, herb for treating, 45. *See* also anthelmintic
Taraxacum spp., 19
tendons and bones, herbs that strengthen, 24,33

testes, inflamed, herbs for treating, 40,59
thiamine. *See* vitamin B1
thirst, herbs for quenching, 18,42,54,66,75,85
throat, dry and uncomfortable, herbs for treating, 55, 87,91. *See* also "hot" and "toxic" conditions
thujone, toxic effects, ix, x
thyme, common and garden, 87
thyme oil, biological effects, 87
thymol, toxic effects, 87
Thymus vulgaris, 87
tight chest. *See* chest, tightness in
tinnitus, herbs for treating, 28,58,60,75,84
tiredness. *See* fatigue
tobacco flavoring, 56
tonic, blood, 21,22,24,28,51,75,76
tonic, brain, 85
tonic, digestive. *See* digestive aid
tonic, general, 1,2,4,8,10,12,15,19,22,24,28,33,34,35, 37,38,40,42,49,51,69,71,77,80,84
tonic, hair, 58,76,78. *See* also hair-growth liniments
tonic, heart. *See* cardiotonic
tonic, male, 14,26,42,76,83
tonic, *qi*, 5,7,10,18,33,51
tonic, *yin*, 58,60,68,75
tooth decay, substances that inhibit, 52
toothache, herbs for treating, 12,35,37,40,63,84, 88
toothpaste, 87
"toxic" conditions. *See* "hot" and "toxic" conditions
trachoma, herb for treating, 35
traditional Chinese medicine, ii
tranquilizing, 59,75,83,85
traumatic injuries, herbs to treat, 9,21,24,38,44,54,78,88
traumatic pain, herb for treating, 44
Trigonella foenum-graecum, 26
triterpenoids: occurrence, 9,15,18,19,30,33, 46, 51,85; biological effects, xiii,30,34,46,52
triterpene acids, occurrence and biological effects, 71,87
triterpene glycosides: occurrence, 5,6,24,44,51, 85; biological effects, 5,24,44. *See* also saponins
triterpene lactones, 19
tuberculosis, pulmonary, herbs for treating, 35, 90,91
tumors. *See* cancer
turmeric, 88,89
Typha species, 9
typhoid, herb for treating, 35
ulcer, duodenal. *See* duodenal ulcer
ulcers, herbs for treating, 35
ulcers, skin. *See* skin ulcers
ulcer, stomach. *See* stomach ulcer
upper respiratory tract infections, herbs to treat, 19,47
urinary tract infections, herb for treating, 19
urination difficulties. *See* dysuria
urination, excessive, herbs for treating, 14,83
urine flow, lack of, herb for treating, 19. *See* also dysuria
ursolic acid, occurrence and biological effects, 52,58,87
urticaria, herbs for treating, 47,54,65,75. *See* also allergies
uterine bleeding, herbs for treating, 5,45,75
uterine inhibitory, 22. *See* also muscle, smooth, relaxant
uterine stimulant, 13,14,22,26,53,72,88. *See* also muscle stimulant
uterine tonic, 81
vaginal tonic, 81
vaginal trichomoniasis, herb for treating, 35
vasodilating, 5,34,45,78
vertigo, herb for treating, 75
Vigna radiata var. *radiata*, 66
viral infections. *See* infections, viral
vision-improving properties, 10,16,58,60
vision, blurred, herbs for treating, 58,60,84
"vital energy." *See qi*
vitamins, xiii
vitamin A, 1,12,20,26,51,72
vitamin B, 20
vitamin B1, 1,16,26,46,49,60,72
vitamin B2, 46,51,60,72
vitamin B6, 1
vitamin B12, 1
vitamin C, 1,9,12,14,20,26,46,51,60,72,90
vitamin D, 20
vitamin E, 1,24,57,72,74
vitamin K, 1
volatile oil: occurrence, 4,7,10,16,18,37,48,53, 64,87; biological effects, 37,53,64,87
vomiting, herb for treating, 40
vomiting blood, herbs for treating, 9,75
warming herbs, 26,42,75
warts, herbs for treating, 10, 49
watercress, iii,55,90
weak knees, herbs for treating, 28,75
weakness, due to loss of blood, herb for treating, 21
weakness, general, herbs to treat, 5,18,28, 33,42,60,77,84
weakness of legs, herb for treating, 24
wet dreams. *See* spermatorrhea
wheezing, herb for treating, 40
wine curing. *See* herb processing
wines, herbs in, 58,74
wound-healing, 2,5,37,38,44,56,65,66,72
wounds, herbs for treating, 2,5,44
wrinkles, cosmetics for, 8,71,77
Wu Shi Er Bing Fang, 70
wumei, 65
wuweizi, 83
xanthotoxin, occurrence and toxicity, 4
yin and *yang*, 42,51
yin tonic. *See* tonic, *yin*
Yin Zhan Zhen Yao (a diet herbal), 85
yiyiren, 49
zhu. *See cangzhu*
Zingiber officinale, 40
Zingiberaceae, 40,88
Ziziphus spp., 51,85
zivulgarin, occurrence and biological effects, 86

NOTES

NOTES

NOTES

NOTES